HEALTHCARE GONE WILD

How We Ruined
Our Healthcare System

GEORGE F. NARYSHKIN, DMD, BS
with BILL KABA, MBA, BS

authorHOUSE®

AuthorHouse™
1663 Liberty Drive
Bloomington, IN 47403
www.authorhouse.com
Phone: 1 (800) 839-8640

Published by AuthorHouse 07/23/2019

ISBN: 978-1-7283-1904-9 (sc)
ISBN: 978-1-7283-1905-6 (hc)
ISBN: 978-1-7283-1903-2 (e)

Library of Congress Control Number: 2019909709

CONTENTS

For my Dad

He loved the experience of life and told me,
"George, life is great."
He always asked me, "Why is that?"
And, "Why do you think that occurs?"
You made me who I am Dad.

PROLOGUE

WHY ARE WE WRITING THIS BOOK?

George

So who am I? Why am I writing this book? And most importantly, why should you read it?

All great questions. My name is George F. Naryshkin. My grandparents immigrated here in the late 1800s and early 1900s from Russia and the Austro-Hungarian Empire (present day Slovakia).

All of my grandparents were "do-it-yourself" survivalists who built their own houses, grew their own food, and raised their own livestock.

In particular, my father's father (Fedor Naryshkin) was a self-educated naturalist who enjoyed reading anything about science. I still have many of his natural history, biology and geology books. Unfortunately, all of them are in Russian.

Fedor influenced my father by giving him a thirst for knowledge. My father worked like a mule his entire life, first attending college to become a teacher, followed by becoming a dentist, and eventually, entering medicine. He retired from a 30+ year career as an OB-GYN. Like his father, he too was a naturalist who also loved farming.

Then comes George F. (me). Both my grandfather Fedor and my father George had a tremendous influence on my quest for the knowledge of how the world works. I became a geologist, completing my senior thesis at Baylor University in 1986 on the Waco Mammoth Site, which still bears the name I gave it, and is now a National Monument. After my undergraduate studies, I worked at an airport in California, learning what I could about aviation while taking flying lessons simultaneously.

I attended Temple University Dental School, graduating in 1986. During my years in Dental School, I was also enrolled in the Air Force ROTC, and I immediately entered UPT (undergraduate pilot training) in Lubbock, Texas at Reese AFB in 1986, part of the class 8707. I deferred starting my career as a dentist in order to learn to fly military aircraft.

I spent 6 years on active duty flying nuclear equipped B-52 G Stratofortress Bombers; I was a nuclear warrior.

My years from 1991 through the present professionally consisted of me working as a dental practitioner, owning two private practices, as well as working in multiple dental franchises and performing contract work in nursing homes, jails, prisons and as a military contractor.

The people who most contributed to my intellectual curiosity involved multiple professors at both Baylor University (geology) and at Temple University (dentistry). Experiences that influenced me include my time as a USAF military pilot, and during the entirety of my dental career, observing the healthcare industry up close.

As a "customer" of the modern Medical Industrial Complex (medical, dental and mental health practitioners, big pharma, insurance companies, medical and dental device companies), I have "consumed" their "product/service" while suffering as an ulcerative colitis, kidney and gall bladder disease patient. As a result of these (and other) experiences, I have a vast history involving searching for the truth while investigating treatments for my conditions.

I am writing this book as an observer of how "we" (government, corporations and *we* consumers of healthcare) have ruined our healthcare system, how our perceptions of medicine and dentistry have been manipulated by the medical industrial complex, and by the willingness of the practitioners to cater to this perception, to work together to produce a very sick system, leading to a sub-optimal quality of life for most Americans.

I do not claim to know more than others, nor to be more correct then others. I am not writing this book to provide solutions to the problems I will be portraying in this book. I simply want to apply my unique point of view to examine what has occurred in the United States that got all of us into this mess, and hopefully, to inspire you to seek your own approach to your healthcare, and to you having the optimal quality of life that you desire and deserve. And while I do claim to have a fair amount of insight into our failures, I do not claim to have the definitive solutions to solve all of our problems.

I am asking you to trust me in this journey we are about to take together. I do not cite all of the research sources discussed in this book; this is not a research paper. I give credit where it is due to researchers when I have their information. All statements and ideas in this book are from my exposure to real research, and you will just have to keep an open mind and try to not simply shut down when you read something that you do not agree with, or that is contrary to what you have been "taught" (in some cases, brainwashed) by the medical industrial complex.

Bill

And who is Bill? I am the patriarch of a family of talented writers and academics in the field of writing. George and I grew up in the same town and shared similar interests throughout our lives. We even attended Rutgers University together.

I am talented in the area of business financial analysis and accounting, working for 35 years in the world of corporate financial planning and analysis, but I am multi-experienced in many science fields. My "education" in science is from reading hundreds of books on science, both the natural and social sciences, anthropology, and philosophy. Thusly, my scientific education is all informal and is driven primarily by intellectual curiosity.

Currently, I am an avid playwright, screenplay writer and novelist, living in Irvine, California, with a few published works, and many more manuscripts waiting in the wings to be published.

George and I share common interests in life; we were members of four different music bands (included concert, stage, marching and rock bands), roomed together on two different occasions, and through our lives discussed topics such as the ones found in this book.

We are also unconventional, nonconformist, outside-the-box thinkers.

George has experience and insight into the medical/dental field while I excel in the communication/writing fields. We decided to collaborate on this work, utilizing the strengths each of us possess in order to communicate this problem that plagues all of us. I am assisting

George on this book for many of the same reasons he started writing it: to apply my unique point of view to examine what has occurred that got us all into this mess, and to hopefully inspire you to seek your own approach to your healthcare so that you can have the optimal quality of life that you desire and deserve.

BIOGRAPHIES

(HOW OUR LIFE EXPERIENCES QUALIFY US TO HAVE AN OPINION ON WHAT IS RUINING OUR HEALTHCARE SYSTEM)

George's Life Experiences

Autopsy Room Assistant

I begin with a morbid subject. At 18 years of age I worked in the morgue at a hospital in my hometown. It was a great introduction to medicine. I observed the dead, I dissected the dead, and I was present during the diagnoses of what made them "the dead". I closed up the dead after the autopsy was completed. I respected the dead.

What I came away with influenced how I look at physicians. I observed patients who died of heart attacks at age 40 with little body fat and no cholesterol in their coronary arteries.

I observed patients who died at 85 with coronary arteries blocked by cholesterol.

I observed an 80-year-old patient who died as a result of having the aorta replaced with artificial blood vessels and died from bleeding out as a result of an operation meant to "save" his life.

This experience served to stimulate my intellectual curiosity, an excellent trait for someone aspiring to become a scientist. We are told that if we exercise and don't eat fat we will extend our life expectancy, and that we will not die of heart failure.

We are told that we must watch our diet or we will die prematurely of heart attack.

We are told that we must fix things that our physician tells us to because it can be done, and we are not provided with a thorough scientific explanation of why we should "fix" whatever is "broken", or about all of our options.

We all die of something. Is there ANY value in describing why you think someone died after age 80, after they have met or exceeded the average life expectancy of a human being? Does it really matter? Does it serve any purpose?

What's wrong with simply stating that the patient died of TIME. This description should suffice.

Geology Student

When I was trained as a geologist at Baylor University, I was taught to observe what I saw, and from those observations, to decide what questions were important to ask in order to gain new insights and knowledge into a specific geological problem. When I uncovered new bones, I did not attempt to regurgitate what others before me had written. I knew what others had accomplished before me through my conducting literature reviews. I simply recorded what I saw and then thought of what questions were important to ask, and what additional research might be of value. I did not assume anything. I did not unnecessarily repeat what others had accomplished before me.

I had very dedicated and disciplined instructors who lived by the rule of recording what we saw, performing necessary experiments, and presenting ALL of the data, as the purpose of our work as scientists was to further knowledge, not prove a point.

We were strenuously questioned in front of our colleagues to make sure that we were able to back up our research and conclusions. We could not (as most scientists do now) simply make blanket statements with no evidence to back up these statements. We were taught that we could not hide behind an agenda.

In a nutshell, we were taught how to be scientists and how to correctly use the scientific method.

Aviator

As a USAF pilot, I trained in an environment in which we were taught to trust those who came before us, as we were not to "decide" what was right or wrong. Engineers and test pilots discovered the limits of the aircraft, and I was asked to memorize them and to fly the aircraft to those limitations. It was not my job to second guess the engineers and test pilots. There was no alternate interpretation of the data. We had inherited the benefit of the application of hundreds of thousands of hours of science involving aeronautics in general, and of testing the capabilities of a specific aircraft.

We did not base our practices or actions on consensus, or a vote. We knew the raw facts, the limits of the aircraft.

Flying didn't have to do with who you knew, or what political party you favored. It was pure, based on what was necessary, what has been proven to be correct. We had the benefit of the experts in the scientific field of aeronautics. I miss my years as a military pilot as it has spoiled me into thinking that the rest of the world communicated and acted in the same way as military pilots, and that period in my life shaped my thought process and is a major reason why I am writing this book.

I equate the work performed by engineers and test pilots which allow our pilots to perform their flying duties with near perfect proficiency to how physicians and dentists should practice medicine and dentistry.

I claim that there are next to no test pilots in medicine anymore. Not so long ago, the test pilots of science correctly carried out scientific experiments and communicated their results. They have disappeared and now our physicians and dentists are left to practice medicine based on fads, political correctness and fear.

Dental School

As a dental student at Temple University Dental School, I was bombarded with millions of bits of information that I was required to memorize and regurgitate on exams. I was also encouraged by my instructors to find better ways to treat patients by experimenting with different techniques.

My professors had a requirement prior to every lecture; to present to their students with five minutes of results that most dentists would say were substandard but which had excellent long lasting results for the patient. We were taught that many of the procedures we performed were done to please an insurance company in order for the school to receive payments from them, but that these results were not necessary to achieve the best result for the patient. As an example, I will use a root canal procedure. Dentists attempt to fill the canals to the tip of the root. This does not determine the long term success of a root canal procedure however. But an insurance company will deny payment to a dentist if the canal does not look filled on an X-ray. Many patients have been put through unnecessary repeat root canal procedures, including surgery through the gums, in order to have the fill appear acceptable to insurance companies. Some even had their perfectly good teeth extracted because an insurance company would not pay to have the tooth crowned if the root canal fill did not look "correct" on an X-ray, even though it could have lasted the patient's lifetime.

Aircraft are standardized. Each one is built as an exact copy of the others. If we know that its engine must have its blades checked or replaced every 100,000 hours, we know this applies to the engines on similar aircraft. And we made sure that we checked it as our lives and the outcome of our mission depended on it.

People are NOT standardized, but your dentist and physician treats you as if you were. That way they can find many things that they must change in you, in order to make you fit a standardized model, something that in reality does not exist.

Author

I have two other published works and one published thesis that have taught me how to collect my thoughts and express them in an efficient manner.

Understanding Why: Evolution, Beliefs and Your Reality, was written to codify my views on why we do what we do, based on evolution, and why the application of the scientific method offers our best hope of solving our problems, be they personal or political, local or global.

In *Healthy? Says Who? The Most Controversial Book You Will Ever Read*, I started to explore the failures of the medical industrial complex. *Healthcare Gone Wild* is a more expansive view of the foundation I built in *Healthy? Says Who?*

My senior thesis was completed at Baylor University in 1980, titled, *The Significance of the Waco Mammoth Site to Central Texas Pleistocene History*. It is now a National Monument.

I will be referencing both of my books throughout this work.

My Medical problems/injuries

Physical injuries I had to overcome: various lacerations, broken rib, dislocated rib, torn Achilles tendon, lower back injury, neck injury, gall bladder (removed), kidney stone (treated), ulcerative colitis that almost killed me (eventually self-treated), hiatal hernia, reattached biceps tendon and Deputren's contracture (surgery).

On Common Ground

One consistency I experienced between dentistry and military aviation involved the optimal protocol for command in control; translation, "Who's in charge?" There is only ONE commander in an aircraft; the pilot. The pilot is in command, and only the commander makes decisions in the aircraft. If the commander is a 2nd Lieutenant, and the navigator a General, the 2nd Lieutenant commands. It is the only way the aircraft can be flown successfully and safely.

The same hierarchy should exist in treating a patient successfully. A new dentist or physician, even one fresh out of school, commands what is done to their patient. Not a nurse or hygienist, even if they have 30 years' experience. And an insurance company should NEVER be calling the shots, especially when they are using the standardized, one size fits all model described above.

Unfortunately (for us), it does not.

Many physicians and dentists have given in to political correctness and incorrectly interpreted that, if they do not consider what a nurse, or medical assistant, or dental assistant wants, including those with decades of experience, that they are somehow not being politically correct or polite. This practice is both incorrect, not to mention potentially dangerous, even lethal.

Bill's Life Experiences

Student/Professional Background

My undergrad degree was in Accounting, which is the language of business. It's a great field to build your business knowledge from. And if you have even above average business acumen, Accounting and Finance are useful in analyzing all aspects of a business. So my "patient" was the company that I worked for, treating everything from a costly, inefficient minor business operation, say, shipping and receiving, (the medical equivalent of a headache), or a product line that is struggling financially (which would equate to a chronic condition), all the way to a failing factory or brand (which would medically represent a fatal condition if left unattended). I added an MBA to my tool kit and became skilled at FP&A (Financial Planning and Analysis). My "medical tests" were Profit and Loss Statements, Balance Sheets, and Cash Flow Statements, and my diagnoses were made via technical studies like Competitive Benchmarks, Item Rationalizations, Strategic Plans, Supply Strategies and hundreds of product initiatives (item launches, price changes, product discontinuations). I also used my analytical abilities in areas outside my business training, including the reformulation of my company's ice cream product line, the creation of a customized pet food product line and I even designed a frozen food factory that delivered product in a bag versus a tray or bowl years before a competitor accomplished this.

I believe that the combination of intellectual curiosity and learning agility opens up an endless supply of possibilities and adventures, and that these traits qualify me to explore areas outside of my core competencies, my sweet spot, where I can offer a fresh perspective on an existing problem that the "experts" are missing out on because they are too invested in their fields.

Writer

After 35+ years working in FP&A, I took a sabbatical to focus on writing. My story telling is through stage plays, screenplays and novels. I tend to also focus on comedy and science fiction, but dabble in drama from time to time. It all stems from an overactive imagination and a desire to communicate my vision to others. When coupled with my strong intellectual curiosity and learning agility tendencies, it is a powerful recipe for communicating new and unorthodox ideas.

Hopefully, this prevails as I help George tell this story to you.

My Medical problems/injuries

Broken bones (mostly fingers and toes), testicular cancer (surgery, radiation therapy), kidney tumor (surgery), inguinal hernia (surgery), tumor removed from popliteal fossa (knee pit, surgery), tumor removed from finger (surgery), herniated disc (micro-surgery), high blood pressure and high cholesterol "diagnoses" (self-treated). Lastly, I suffer from a very rare eye condition called Pellucid Marginal Degeneration (PMD); my corneas are misshapen. As a result, I see the world much the way you would if you were at a 3D movie and lifted up the 3D glasses; I see multiple copies of everything. Fortunately, I can correct it with very expensive scleral contact lenses, custom made to fit my eye. Unfortunately, these lenses are not covered by any medical insurances, even my very expensive plan, so my out of pocket costs are $7,000 every time I need new lenses.

THE PURPOSE OF THE BOOK?

(SO JUST WHAT IS THE PROBLEM?)

Why are we taking both your and our time in writing this book?

We are writing this book because we have become frustrated with what goes on in our medical and dental professions as they are practiced in the medical industrial complex. Our concept of reality has been hijacked by doctors and politicians. And it doesn't help matters that the media, including (maybe especially) the Internet, also exacerbates the problem.

Christopher Hitchens, in *god is not Great,* wrote that religion exists because people fear death, and religion takes anxiety away from the believer. Now, the medical industrial complex has replaced religion by offering the public immortality if they just follow their rules. This, however, is not the case.

In the past, we passed information along that was created from well planned and executed scientific research projects. A lot of time went into these projects, and they were planned with great care as the person carrying out the research only had so much time to dedicate to a project. They then replayed their research project to be sure they recorded all the data correctly, and that what they described was exactly what they did, and that a reader of their research could repeat the study and come up with the exact same results. The results underwent a process known as peer review in the scientific community, and if they passed this high level of scrutiny, they were inspected by a prospective publisher who would also investigate the claims of the author of the research before publishing.

The publisher would ask to see the original idea of the research (what question was the researcher attempting to answer), then look at all of the patient records (if the author claimed 1,000 patients participated in the study, do they have those records to prove it?). The reviewer would read perhaps 10% of arbitrarily selected records to be sure the records were kept correctly. They then would personally interview perhaps another 10% of the patient participants to validate the written records.

They would look at all data, records and personal interviews and then sit down to see if the method was logical, and if the sequence of events recorded were sensible in attempting to answer the original question.

Did it make sense? Were the patients chosen correctly? Was there a correct amount of a control group (patients who did not participate in the study but were willing to be observed)?

Were the dependent and the independent variables limited to one?

If the parameters of the study claimed to follow a patient from age 10 to 30, did it? Or did the researcher simply project his idea of what the results should be when the patients reached the age of thirty, but did not actually observe this?

In summary, did the research actually follow the scientific method?

Now let me give you an example of what passes as research today. There are many so called "studies" on the subject of blood pressure. Many claim to have thousands of patients in their study when in fact they either exaggerated the amount of subjects, or simply read another published paper and included those patients in their study. They then "project" what they think should happen as a patient ages into their results. They claim that by using their blood pressure medicine to lower blood pressure, the patients will live longer. These results never occurred as the paper only covered a two year period, not long enough to evaluate an increase in longevity. But the author feels it is ok because who would question him? Or maybe the results of the study provides answers that the reader (often, someone that might financially benefit from the results, say, a pharmaceutical company!) is seeking.

This last comment offers a perfect example of research creating a market for a product; blood pressure medication.

The truth is, longevity is not increased with the use of any blood pressure lowering drug, or by lowering blood pressure by any means (more on this subject later).

But no one investigated these results when they were published online by a publisher who was only interested in how many times the story was viewed. Or by how much Big Pharma could increase its bottom line and drive up its stock value.

If more viewers choose one story over another, the most chosen would move to the top of the search list, making it more and more difficult to find less "popular" articles. It has also been noted by others that scientists who produce real research publish their articles in obscure journals that only their colleges would be interested in reading.

And as most of us have seen, the most popular articles are the ones that follow fads, or have an exciting or appealing title, or that manipulate our human predisposition to seek stories that scare us, as our prehistoric ancestors were more likely to survive and thrive (create copies of themselves) if they were cognizant of as many dangers in their surroundings as possible.

One more example of what exactly is "the problem." It will be delved into further, but here is a tease.

We all know about the Holocaust and the tragic fate of those executed in the camps, and the horrible conditions that the survivors were subject to.

Would you be surprised to find out that the survivors, on average, had longer life expectancies (seven years longer) than a "control" group of Jewish peoples that were born around the same time (both groups were born between 1911 and 1945) that were living in what would become the state of Israel after World War II? And that the survivors had significantly higher rates of "chronic" conditions (obesity, cancer, hypertension to name just a few) and still outlived the control group?

These two results fly in the face in all that we have been told by the medical industrial complex.

DISCLAIMER

We are not promoting anything in this book; we are simply stating the facts. I do not know if using any of the substances or following the practices discussed in this book prolongs life, but they certainly do not reduce life span. Maybe reducing stress can help us live longer, but "stress", like the word "healthy", really has no definition. Is it chemical stress? Physical stress? Mental stress? And how is it measured?

We do not know.

This book is not meant as a medical manual, so please do not interpret it as one. Only YOU can decide what to do with your body. We are not giving you advice on what you should do medically with your body.

Warning; the views found in this book may come across as being blunt and insensitive. The reader is already going to be discombobulated and flummoxed as you discover all the misinformation that the medical industrial complex, the media, and big government has been disseminating. Please do not let our approach contribute to the depletion of your emotional capital; the previously stated villains have already spent your whole life doing this! But the reason for our frankness is because part of the reason why we are in this mess is because we all are too politically correct and we are too afraid to hurt other people's feelings. We don't challenge our healthcare providers, we don't question the "evidence" that they are using to treat us, and we all want to be liked.

Fortunately (or perhaps, unfortunately!) for you, the authors of this work don't care if we are unpopular as a result of this work. Actually, we fully expect to ruffle a lot of feathers. We expect a lot of angry doctors, dentists, psychotherapists, drug and insurance companies, and politicians to be unhappy with this book. But hopefully, you will realize that we are writing this to entertain and enlighten you.

FOUNDATIONS

I want to begin this chapter by first letting you know that I have met and have been treated by some excellent physicians and dentists. I have also met many physicians and dentists who inspired me to write this book. Unfortunately, most of the physicians and dentists I have encountered do not practice medicine and dentistry the way it should be practiced. They are a large part of why our healthcare system has gone wild.

DEFINITIONS

Health, fitness and other misunderstood terms

I had to put this topic in the front of this book as this is an area of confusion and a major source of problems that we have with our healthcare system today.

Health (not what most people think)

The dictionary definition of health is a "sense of well-being". So basically, it is a "feeling" or psychological state of mind. The modern definition of health is "the state of being free from illness or injury." Healthy is defined as "not diseased." The World Health Organization (WHO) defines health as "the state of complete physical, mental, and social wellbeing and not merely the absence of disease or infirmity." In either sense, health is a state of action that includes prevention, care, and individual responsibility to achieve optimal health.

The modern re-defining of "health" was by WHO in 1984; the U.S. redefinition occurred in 2010. The medical industrial complex redefines the term "health" on a continual basis by creating "problems" (illnesses) where they don't exist.

Think about all those TV commercials where the announcer states that their food or vitamins are a "healthy" choice. What does that mean to you? I think most viewers would interpret that statement to mean that you will live longer if you consume their product.

When the statement "healthy" is used by a person, what it really means is that the owner of the product thinks that if you consume their product you will "feel" better. And sometimes that claim might be correct. However, the companies or owners of the products find that it sells better if they put it into a vague category of "healthy" claims. And they don't receive retaliation from consumers as most consumers want to think that consuming these product does make you live longer.

When I tried to find a medical definition of the word "health," I only found one from the 1930's. I no longer have the reference, but researchers who carried out an experiment on longevity in mice used it in this way: if an organism lives longer than the general population of genetically similarly animals with less major illness (heart disease, diabetes, cancer) then, that animal is said to have better health than the rest of the population.

You will discover as you read on that no one uses the word "health" correctly. Americans use the word health when they mean to use the word "fit" or "fitness."

Good health is something many people wish existed. It is a fantasy.

The Food and Drug Administration (FDA), as of the publishing of this book, has not come up with a definition of "healthy." They are only concerned with the term for "proper" food labeling.

Fitness

A more confusing definition, but it has to do with the ability of an organism to pass its genetic material on to its offspring. (Europeans use the term to describe a person's ability to use their body; if a soccer player sprains his ankle, he is not fit, but he is healthy, as he is not sick.)

Most Americans use fitness and healthy interchangeably, and this causes much of the confusion in our healthcare system. Which is exactly what big government and the medical industrial complex want to happen; if we are distracted and confused, we won't notice the beating that we're taking.

Longevity

What can be done to increase our time on Earth? Very few studies refer to actual research. The best example of scientific research is a study on mice which has been reproduced all over the world with different species of mammals, always yielding the same results. A period of starvation in mammals increases the average length of life by 33%, and the species will experience 50% less major illness (cancers, diabetes and heart disease).

Recently, Amanda Ruggeri published what appears to be an academic historical account of human longevity based on anthropological and literary evidence. The conclusion: human longevity has not increased in 10,000 years. In fact, in ancient England, where records were kept of date of birth and death, the wealthy had shorter life spans than the poor.

The above holds true today, as studies performed correctly and which do not attempt to give in to political correctness, find that access to medical treatment and money do not determine length of life.

What has changed since 10,000 years ago is that the "median" age of humans has increased, meaning, a higher percentage of humans make it to middle age. But the ultimate age that a human can achieve has not increased with all that science has to offer.

Some vaccines have been shown to decrease early death for specific illnesses (1 billion lives saved), blood transfusions (another billion), anti-biotics (200 million), and the bifurcated needle (130 million), were all major medical breakthroughs that saved lives, but did nothing to extend human longevity. And non-medical breakthroughs did just as much to save lives, with inventions such as toilets (1 billion lives saved), synthetic fertilizers (another billion), pasteurization (250 million) and water chlorination (175 million). But the largest overall advances leading to increased life expectancies (and to our current quality of life) were not medical or non-medical advances and inventions; they were the result of capitalism. Events like the industrial revolution. Starting with England, followed by Western Europe, North America and East Asia, and now transforming the developing world into the developed world in the last 50 years, mostly due to the transition from Communism (Russia, Eastern Europe, China and Vietnam) to Capitalism, and driving accessibility to the previously stated breakthroughs. Another event causing increases in life expectancies occurred right after World War II. The Marshall Plan/United Nations/WTO-IMF-World Bank basically created the modern world in terms of finance, industrialization and trade, rebuilding Europe and Japan, creating the rules for countries to cooperate with each other, and discouraging participating countries from ever going to war with one another, leading to exponential improvements in quality of life and life expectancies on Earth. And even though this infrastructure lead to the Cold War, which almost destroyed the planet, it prevailed in the long run, causing Communism to fail and Capitalist Democracies to flourish.

Stress

There is a lot of discussion about stress these days. I tend to approach the subject by looking at stress in the context of the animal kingdom, of which, human beings are a member. That's right, we are just another animal among eight million species of animals, or, more specifically, 300 species of primates.

Consider pre-agricultural man walking down a path to the watering hole. Out of nowhere, a saber-toothed tiger appears. The human is instantly in a stressful situation, prompting their body to react. Adrenaline flows in massive quantities, their senses are in a heightened alert mode; it's fight or flight time.

The human that survives the encounter returns to the tribe and eventually (hopefully) procreates, allowing their superior survivability traits to be passed on to the gene pool. The human that dies (hopefully before they reproduced) does not. What's more, the stress disappears once they are back amongst tribe mates.

This would be called "good" mental stress. (Providing you lived and did not suffer long term PTSD from the encounter!) This kind of stress might add to longevity.

So what is the definition of stress? The textbook definition of stress is "a state of mental or emotional strain or tension resulting from adverse or very demanding circumstances."

We do not know how to measure stress nor to equate it to this definition when we say "stress", nor its effect on illness or longevity. It is simply "stated."

Nutrition

During WWII, many unfortunate humans were kept in poor living conditions, and received little or no food. Those who were starved for a prolonged timed died as a result. Some of those that were starved but did not die lived into their hundreds.

What do all your nurses, physicians, friends and favorite TV personalities tell you about food? They all tell us that we need good "nutrition" in order to live long, "healthy" lives. What are they all talking about? If you were to describe the "nutrition" of the prisoners of WWII, but not tell your audience who they were, what would they say? They would tell you that they are on a "dangerous" diet, that they will get cancer and other scary sounding diseases and conditions, and that they will surely die young.

Their idea of "nutrition" is warped as they think you must have "good nutrition", which apparently means, "eat a lot of things we say are good", and "don't eat things we say are NOT good."

So, were the WWII prisoners receiving "good" nutrition? Or were they "malnourished?"

Science (the internet has made us all much dumber)

Most of the problems that we face in the world today are due to people not being able to communicate properly with one another. Many of these miscommunications are in the field of science.

I attended dental school from 1982 to 1986. My wise instructors lectured us students many times on their frustration with the observation that students enrolled in science disciplines were becoming less and less able to distinguish between an agenda driven paper and a valid research paper.

So......what is science? I am not going to give you a dictionary definition. I will explain it this way. Science "is a way of living your life", (*Understanding Why, Evolution, Beliefs and Your Reality*, Naryshkin). It is a way of making sense of the world around you, of the universe. Your understanding is shaped by people questioning how the universe works, then planning a study to prove or disprove their idea. The researcher does not eliminate data that does not agree with their original thoughts on what the outcome of the study might show.

Proper scientific experimentation: a scientist has an idea of how something in our universe works. (This is what is known as a hypothesis). They define what they are attempting to find out, design how they will go about doing this, and present all of the data and findings, then state what the data shows. There must be only ONE variable in a properly carried out study.

What is being labeled as "science" these days: a person (I cannot refer to them as a scientist) states an idea (maybe), then states how they will go about performing their research or collecting data. They then remove data that does not agree with their desired outcome and redefine the original idea in order to fit the data. They have an agenda, namely, to prove that their original idea was correct. They are *not* undertaking their project to further our understanding of our universe.

An example of this follows. A drug company wants to show that its new drug (drug M) lowers blood pressure in men. They state that they will collect data from arbitrary cardiac patients and present it.

While collecting their data, they find that only men in the age group 60-65 had slightly lower blood pressure after taking drug M; drug M had no effect on every other age group. Rather than presenting all of the data which would demonstrate that drug M does not work as thought, they delete all data except for men in the 60-65 age group, then restate the paper to indicate that it was only meant to study men in the age group 60-65 and, voila, they offer "proof" that drug M lowers high blood pressure!

Their findings will insure that the drug company will continue to fund their research lab. Very few if any readers will ask to see all of their data, or ask to and be allowed to interview any of the patients that participated in the "research."

In order to perform proper research, the researcher must define the parameters of the study (does it involve humans of all ages and races?), the amount of time that the study will cover, the variables (the things that the researcher will alter in the study), and the uncontrollable variables (the things that the researcher cannot control, such as if the subjects are to eat only fruit every day for one year, how can the researcher be sure that they really did only eat fruit)?

If the study is to help in determining whether or not a procedure or drug increases the patient's longevity, did they actually study the subject until they died?

Did the researcher inform the reader of how many subjects they included in the study, and how many did not complete the entire study, and why? Did they inform the reader of the whereabouts of the subject's records and provide access to them? Are they willing to have a valid researcher examine their research and subjects before and after publishing? Was the study peer reviewed?

Controlling the variables is probably the most important factor in conducting proper research, yet it is ignored by most "researchers."

When, for example, a researcher conducts a study on longevity and does not name the variable that they will control and manipulate, they have designed an improper research environment.

The famous rodent study from the 1930's kept mice from birth to death in an isolated cage. The researcher was able to control everything that the animals ate and drank for their entire life, and only varied the amount of food, not the type of food, that the subjects were fed. In this instance, it was crystal clear what was being studied, and the controlled variable was easily verified.

Most modern papers labeled as "research" are simply essays on how a human responds to a questionnaire. The variable was not controlled as the human subjects travelled where they wanted to, ate what they wanted to, and lived as they pleased. The questionnaires did nothing to verify even if what they remembered was true.

Now most physicians, dentists, and mental health professionals justify their practices on what their colleagues think. They prioritize consensus over science. They believe that what is most important in what they diagnose, or treatment plan is what their friends will think is correct, over what science demonstrates.

Associations (Correlation and Causation)

"When ice cream sales increase, there is an increase in drowning deaths. Therefore, ice cream consumption may cause death by drowning."

This is an example of the statistical concept that correlation does not imply causation; sometimes, the connection is a result of coincidence and/or a third variable. In this case, the third variable is temperature. People go swimming when the temperature is higher. They also consume more ice cream when it is warmer. Associating drowning with ice cream consumption is a bad association.

Much of bad research is the result of assumptions rather than just reading the data. Sometimes the assumptions turn out to be the incorrect interpretation of associations.

Some misinformed scientists make statements such as "some animals, after living in caves, have become blind since they did not need their sight." It is true that the animal doesn't have sight. It is true that the animal lives in a cave with no light. The untrue statement is that the animal's blindness was caused by the lack of light. This suggests that the environment somehow changes genetics to take advantage of that environment, or that the lack of something tells the genetic material to remove something from the animals DNA.

The reality is that animals always have genetic mutations. If these mutations benefit the animal, it prospers and reproduces at a higher rate than the animals without that mutation. So in the above example, the darkness does not cause the loss of site. An animal with a genetic mutation of no sight will not know they are in a lightless environment, they reproduce, and this mutation is carried on. Animals without the mutation will seek light and escape, or will not reproduce as they are not happy, not being able to see. (This is what Charles Darwin described in his Theory of Evolution and Natural Selection).

In medicine, remarks are made such as, "People who exercise into late life live longer." This makes logical sense to most people. The reality could be that people with the genetic mutation for long life feel better (are more fit) in their older age, so they are more active. In fact, studies have shown that aerobic exercise lessens longevity in humans.

Cardio exercises increase your chance of heart attack and premature death if done after age 40. More on this later.

Another good example to explain correlation and causation involves Cuba, where aging population studies have shown that Cuba has one of the highest stable genetic populations and the oldest living population in the world. When filling out questions on their daily habits, most of the centenarians noted that they smoke at least one cigar a day and drink one cup of coffee a day. Is this a biological association? Or is it political? Perhaps citizens of Cuba feel obligated to say they smoke one cigar a day since Cuba is famous for their cigars. This might be a study of how Cubans respond to health questionnaires rather than on what gives them their longevity.

So, you see, associations might not be properly interpreted. I am sure many times they are. But many times in medicine, combined with their lack of ability to discern science, information is not interpreted correctly.

40 years ago, the potential for tobacco to cause cancer was questioned. I still do not know if the association was properly interpreted. I was taught that it was the heat from the cigarettes that caused the cancer. Recently a report (not research) claimed an association with hot tea and oral cancer. Is it the "heat" of the tea that causes the cancer? Or is it an ingredient in the tea? Did the authors test distilled hot water in the report? Or was the report based on a questionnaire that the subjects simply had to answer about what they drank?

Research has to be correctly carried out and clearly communicated to the reader in order for it to be meaningful.

So political groups, special interest groups and others, both ignorant people and those that don't understand the scientific method, will read a "report", interpret it as "research", and run with it. They will write editorials and fill the internet with this questionable information, and millions will bite on it and receive it as gospel.

The medical industrial complex is more focused on "reports" than "research." They are largely ignoring the scientific method. They have turned medicine into a "soft science", like economics or sociology. This is the root cause of our healthcare system's metamorphosis. Healthcare professionals used to be scientists that were experts at medicine, or dentistry, or mental healthcare. Now they are nothing more than practitioners of soft science.

Various and Sundry Terminology

Lastly, some nonsensical words and phrases that are used in fake scientific articles:

"Not exactly", and "not sure" are meaningless and attempt to make the reader think the evidence shown is highly reliable when the correct words should be "I don't know" when defining their "evidence."

"Studies" referenced by journalists only refer to questionnaires, not data. And most published "studies" are not even researched at all. A journalist decides that the Japanese live the longest without actually looking at the data, decides that this is due to their diet, then they visit a Japanese restaurant, or ask a few Japanese people what they eat, and, "voila", they have a "research" paper.

The longest living individuals in various countries were asked what they did that contributed to their longevity. The most common statement I have observed is that they participated in at least one habit every day. The most common habit I have observed is the daily use of tobacco.

Most of us would question this as we are taught tobacco is bad for us, that it causes cancer. What is the truth? Is the questionnaire flawed? Is the Western world flawed? Maybe the war on tobacco is just a political one?

My own observation around tobacco use is that humans have always sought out a way, or a substance, that alters their reality in a pleasant way. Tobacco is one of those substances. Even some non-human animals seem to seek out mind altering substances that they find a benefit in. That statement poses another set of problems. What is relaxation and how do we measure it? Are the participants in the questionnaires influenced by how the questions are phrased? And how much is too much?

Another common trait among the longest living humans is that they did not receive ANY medical care, let alone "regular checkups", throughout their entire life.

Some analysis based on real data:

During WWII, many European Jews were held captive in prison camps with no medical care, and little food or water. They were basically starved to death. It was a cruel time in human history. After the war, our so called medical "experts" predicted that the survivors would all die early deaths due to their treatment, or lack of "nutrition."

Much to everyone's surprise, these survivors had one of the longest life spans of a collective genetic pool of humans. A significant amount of their population lived to be over 100 years old!

How could this happen? The "experts" were stunned due to their ignorance and failure to learn from the past. The studies on mice in the 1930's clearly documented this occurrence. Studies of early humans from over 10,000 years ago demonstrated that some of us lived to be over 100 years old. I am sure we were starving then as well.

In the early 2000's, another "researcher" documented centenarians living in Cuba. They were given a questionnaire on their diets and their habits, and the only similarity among the majority was that they smoked at least one cigar a day and drank at least one cup of coffee a day.

What does your doctor ask you at every appointment? They take your blood pressure and tell you that tobacco and caffeine are bad for you. So was the questionnaire given to the Cubans flawed? Or is the advice you pay good money to your physician for incorrect? And prior to the publishing of this book, yet another government agency reported that drinking up to 25 cups of coffee a day did no harm. How did the authors come up with this information? What does "no harm" mean?

I love this conundrum! I like to question what is "real" and what is the "truth?"

I would guess that Cubans are not able to indulge in a lot of food, and maybe it has become part of their culture to get by on little food. Perhaps they have unknowingly copied the occurrence of the European Jews and the mice in the rodent study.

The coffee and cigars might be insignificant. These substances might actually be providing "a sense of well-being" that would benefit the user.

Ronald Reagan had a way with words. He noted the following about his opposition political party; "They are not stupid, they just know a lot of what is not." That statement can well describe current physicians and their patients.

A HISTORY LESSON

(ARE WE TALKING CONSPIRACY HERE?)

Where did it all go wrong?
Why did it all go wrong?

Bio Plausibility (the Mr. Potato Head syndrome)

I came across an article by a very informed journalist, David Epstein; *When Evidence Says No, But Doctors Say Yes* (*The Atlantic*, February 22, 2017).

In this article, Epstein looks at real research and reveals that many of the medical procedures performed on patients have been proven to not offer them any tangible benefits, yet most physicians will tell a patient that they "need" the procedure in order to live a normal life, meaning longevity. I believe he coined the phrase "bio plausible." He states that it means that if a procedure makes sense to a physician, such as opening a clogged pipe should make liquids flow more freely in them, and if it can be visualized in a biological situation, such as in a patient's heart, they will perform the procedure even if the evidence demonstrates that it does not benefit the patient.

Another bio plausible procedure that does not benefit anyone is that of lowering blood pressure (BP). Two very well executed studies by cardiologists (heart specialists) both concluded that lowering blood pressure from what is widely accepted as high levels does not benefit a patient; it neither provides patients with longevity nor reduces their probability of dying from heart attack or stroke. Additionally, they found that lowering BP after a stroke actually increases the patient's chances of dying from a more massive stroke sooner than if you had not been given BP lowering meds.

To pile onto the ignorance that exists today amongst physicians due to myths and corruption, a medical society recently released a statement saying patients should classify high BP as 120/80 or higher, rather than 140/80, even though data demonstrates that lowering BP doesn't benefit a patient.

When the publicized recommendation for BP was 140/90, more than 50% of all US citizens fell into this category, meaning that those who supported the 140/90 levels were saying that over 50% of one species (us) requires treatment in order to live a normal life.

The newly publicized numbers suggest perhaps 75% of all of us have a condition which needs immediate treatment and medication.

In the UK, a medical organization carried out real research whose objective was to find out if coronary by-pass surgery actually worked. The physicians took a pool of 1,000 prospective patients who were diagnosed with narrowing of the coronary arteries (the blood vessels that feed the heart) and who were experiencing heart pain as a result. These patients were prescribed a procedure where blood vessels from another part of the patient's body were sewn into place where the narrowed arteries were removed.

The variable was kept to ONE. The patients received all the same experience as the others EXCEPT that 50% had the actual blood vessel replacement, and 50% did not. They all were treated as surgical patients, receiving blood work, medicine, general anesthesia, incisions, and sutures.

The results: NO DIFFERENCE in outcome. Coronary by-pass surgery was proven to be a placebo operation. The drugs and relief that you received in a supposed lifesaving operation were enough to relax the patient and eliminate the heart pains.

Explanation as to why it does not work: the heart will develop a new blood supply by the branching off of the blood vessels suppling the heart when existing blood vessels start struggling to do the job. Heart pains are from inflammatory molecules in the body, not lack of oxygen.

When this data was presented in a lecture to a group of heart surgeons who were asked if they agreed with the results, they all raised their hands.

When asked who would still perform the procedure on their patients, a surprising 50% of surgeons raised their hands. When these surgeons were asked to justify their decisions, they explained that if they did not provide the patient with this operation, and when they eventually died (as we all will), their family will sue them for not doing all they could have done.

So what we have been told is a necessary medical procedure is actually "fraud".

When a patient chooses to go for a medical check-up, it should be a "check" up. This means the physician is "checking" how you compare to others. But who are these "others?"

In grade school, we took mental and physical "tests" to measure us against "others." The others were our equals.

Shouldn't a patient also be measured against *their* equals? The physicians first pull the wool over our eyes by saying blood pressure is important and you will die if you don't lower it. But "what" are they measuring you against? Medical journals will say that more than 50% of adults have high blood pressure. Really? What are they comparing you too? If they are comparing you to adults in your age range, then you are "normal." But the stories and essays that are passed on as being "research" don't seem to want to explain this apparent lack of attention to this problem.

We all die. A physician's chart of you simply records the slow deterioration of a human being. It is what happens. They want you to believe that this deterioration is abnormal and is meant to be fixed or changed by the physician and all that medicine has to offer.

I am not aware of any properly conducted research which supports the current conventional "wisdom" among pill pushing physicians, so I can only conclude that it must be a conspiracy being carried out by the medical industrial complex and the politicians that benefit from it through contributions, namely, most of congress. (According to OpenSecrets.org, the third largest interest group contributing to congressional incumbents were Health Professionals, contributing to 52% of all Democrats and 47% of all Republicans, and the 11th largest contributor was Big Pharma, contributing to 46% of all Democrats and 54% of all Republicans. Coming in at number 30 and 32 were

Nurses/Nursing Homes and Health). This decision to lower BP benefits the drug companies, physicians, and politicians. Guess who it doesn't benefit? The "patient."

Christopher Hitchens, author of *god is Not Great*, observed that educated scientists will back up things they learned as children, rather than back up things that they have learned subsequently that go against those things, or their beliefs. This completely contradicts the fundamental teachings of science!

Mr. Potato Head......hmm. Ok, I'll tell you what I mean by this reference. The Mr. Potato Head toy that we all played with as kids consists of a real or plastic potato that comes with multiple body parts which you can substitute for other parts, inserting them and removing them from the potato. Arms, ears, nose, legs, mouths; you get the picture.

Human biology (just like most of the animal kingdom) does not allow this. What I am trying to communicate is that if a cancerous lung is removed from a patient, all lung tissue was not removed from the body. But in the Mr. Potato Head, that would occur.

For example, performing colonoscopies, including polyp removal, does not increase your chances of living a long life. The reason? Cancer does not begin in the tip of a polyp, but its removal has bio plausibility.

Removing a woman's breast does not ensure that she will not die of breast cancer.

Unfortunately for us "patients", medical insurance corporations and legal professions conspire to advance this treatment. As a result, the patient thinks that they must have this procedure done, and that they will live forever if they have polyps removed. (The same thinking holds true for growths removed from lungs and breasts, but more on this later).

The medical industrial complex makes more money if they perform these procedures on you, so they justify their actions as they are decreasing the chance of you suing them in the instance that you die of an intestinal problem rather than of a condition that another specialist group is responsible for. Furthermore, insurance company's profits are a function of their "sales", the amount of insurance that they sell. And while they make higher profits when their sales (premiums) exceed their costs (payments made to medical practitioners, big pharma, medical device companies, etc.), they still benefit if they allow more and more procedures to be treated, providing that they build them into their premiums ahead of time. And while their profit margins are not unusually high as most business go (they range from 3 to 8% of sales), their dollar profits have risen dramatically since the passing of the Affordable Care Act (the top six companies saw an 8.5% increase in the second quarter of 2017, and their stock values have doubled since 2014!) Once a procedure represents a larger portion of their expenditures, they tend to pressure physicians and big pharma to lower costs, which usually result in lower service to you, the customer/patient.

Where do the lawyers come in? A jury consisting of an uneducated and/or misinformed American (your peers; translation, possibly YOU!) can easily be swayed by any argument based on bio plausibility. Jurors love to pay out other people's money, and while they are usually correct in their verdict surrounding lawsuits involving hanky-panky on the part of the medical industrial complex, excessive awards of damages primarily serve to drive up health insurance premiums and make lawyers rich.

How We Devolved From Broke-Fix It to Health Maintenance Coverage (Insurance Misconceptions and Lawyers)

Health Insurance; how did this come about? This is the first, and most significant conspiracy causing healthcare to go wild.

Prior to the 1940's we did not have insurance for medical or dental treatment.

Suddenly, a number of factors coalesced in the 1940's to create the heath "insurance" industry involving unions, government regulation, and businesses. Before World War II, people went to their physician when they had something seriously wrong with them (a broken bone, a laceration that was causing severe blood loss, a sudden illness like food poisoning); when they were "broken." Of course, there were hypochondriacs among us (and still are), that rushed to the doctors with every little ache and pain, believing that they were going to die (we will all eventually die). Patients (they had not become "customers" yet) paid cash for an exam and possibly received medication. The world got along just fine.

1940 comes along and the unions introduce a new concept to us: Medical Insurance. Why did we need insurance to see a physician? The unions wanted to gain members and could not offer more money as they had squeezed as much as they could from the corporations already, some of whom had been exploiting workers, but most of whom were already paying higher wages since demand for workers had increased due to WWII and the end of the Great Depression, and the labor market had shrank due to 16 million Americans going off to fight the war. They invented medical insurance solely to attract members. They offered medical insurance to its members, at a time when no one had it. This was exacerbated by government regulations that arose in the years following World War II, when the U.S. economy was overheating, having emerged from the Great Depression when industry was cranking out hardware to fight the war. The government was worried about inflation (it was double digit for the first few years following WWII), so they placed wage freezes to keep that component of the cost of goods and services from getting out of control. Insurance companies approached all companies, not just unionized ones, and pitched one of their lesser known products, medical insurance. By offering new employees medical insurance, companies found a way to become more attractive, since they couldn't do it through wages. The insurance was free to the employees and cheap to the companies (healthcare costs were under 5% of GDP (Gross Domestic Product) before WWII, versus 17% today!) Unions took advantage of this perk and started exploiting it immediately.

It was a brilliant idea as it made unions seem more attractive to workers. "Join us and we will pay for your medical and dental bills". In order to incentivize physicians and dentists to accept these new insurance products, the unions fabricated an artificial checkup time frame of six months. It was easy to remember, and this assured that the physician would receive a guaranteed income as the insurance companies paid their office every six months for exams, and other small billable procedures that their newly created customers were consuming! And what patient would say no to something that was free, or cost them close to nothing? Soon, physicians and dentists told their patients they should make use of their insurance since it was free. Sadly, this conspiracy exists to present time.

The now "standard" six month dental exam and yearly physical was never based on medicine or science. It exists only because brilliant union leaders, insurance companies, businesses, and politicians had an idea on how to make the workplace more attractive.

And now....no one wants to let go of it. The ACA for all intents and purposes, is on its way to becoming the third rail in American politics, just like Social Security. (The third rail is a reference the New York Subway System, where the third rail provides power to the train and will electrocute anyone that touches it; politicians will not dare go near Social Security, and the ACA is rapidly approaching a similar status). Most people think insurance is necessary for a person to have a tooth repaired or to prevent their impending death. But we do not have insurance to repair our cars (other than for auto accidents), or to have them checked, or to purchase new tires. Could you imagine if we had this type of insurance for everything in our lives? So why do we accept medical and dental insurance to be a "necessity?" All other insurances that we purchase cover catastrophes. In reality, what we refer to as health insurance is actually a health *maintenance* plan. And even if you purchase maintenance for a product, like your car, there are limits placed on what you can ask for it to cover. You can't talk your mechanic into putting on new tires when your existing tires have plenty of tread remaining on them. You are giving your money, and freedom of choice, to a third party who usually does not have the same intention in mind as you in using your money.

A doctor can talk you into taking meds or having procedures done because they believe that you need them based on their cursory examination of you every year.

It is a political tool used to win the votes of uneducated and/or misinformed voters. Proponents of big government study human behavior and are good at manipulating the average citizen into thinking they are in danger if they do not count on big brother to take care of them. They want you to be insecure and to think that you need what your neighbor has, so vote for us.

Big government has found their goose that lays the golden egg, and that egg is our insecurity about our life. They promise to keep us from aging, from losing our teeth, from getting any age related conditions, and ultimately, to keep us from dying. The medical industrial complex has, in fact, replaced our belief in religion with a belief in all of the bull that they are selling us.

And the physicians and dentists happily climb on board for the free ride.

Additionally, insurance companies put fear into patients and physicians, as do lawyers. Attorneys make money by winning law suits. To do this, they must convince a patient that a physician or dentist did them wrong. Then they must put the suggestion that there was wrongdoing on the part of the physician in the form of a lawsuit, and the physician's insurance company feels pressured into settling with the attorney, thus avoiding having to take the case to a court where the attorney will ask for significantly more money.

If the case does go to court, the attorney must convince a jury that the physician did wrong. It can be anything, from not washing their hands, to not documenting what they did or said to the patient. The attorney will do everything possible to get the jury to question the physician's abilities; their job is to manipulate the jury of uneducated and misinformed layman into giving away large sums of money to their client, portraying them as a "victim" of "malpractice." And because America has an over abundance of lawyers (the U.S. has 3.3 lawyers for every 1,000 people, compared to Germany with 1.7 and France with 0.7! Compare that to our 2.3 doctors per 1,000 people, and Germany and France's at 3.4! Or that we have more lawyers then doctors!) There are thousands of legal cases each year. The lawyer's client may well be a victim, but the real victim is the rest of us, who are paying more for healthcare premiums because of the high cost of malpractice insurance that doctor's must pay because of America's oversupply of lawyers and the litigious nature of our citizenry.

The fear of not dotting all the i's and crossing all the t's is why some physicians perform the countless exams and tests on each patient. And if you do not give them permission, they must document that they warned you that you might have one or more deadly diseases, but that you would not allow them to search for them.

These practices give the physician permission to use the "what if" phrase over and over again.

It's a conspiracy, as all of the above nonsense is not necessary, but all parties involved, with the exception of the PATIENT, benefit financially from this arrangement of fear mongering and the need for thorough documentation.

Everything is a problem!

In the 1970's, normal blood pressure was listed as 179/98 by whatever organization the government allowed to be in charge of such a thing. It was not until the discovery of medications that could lower your blood pressure that the "normal" reading was changed. This helped pharmaceutical companies, physicians, attorneys and insurance companies. Oh, and politicians. And it "supposedly" helped the "patient."

Now your senator or congressman tells you that *they're* going to fight to get *your* insurance company to pay for regular blood pressure check-ups, and to pay for medication. It was a win-win situation for everyone involved EXCEPT FOR YOU!

Addiction to alcohol and drugs? Now this is considered to be a medical condition and results in the same thing as blood pressure being lowered. It is big business to treat drug addiction. Build a house, put a bunch of addicts in it, and charge $20,000/month for each "patient" to sit it in a room and talk to each other. Of course, a physician must monitor this and receives big bucks to be on site.

Politicians want anything and everything to be treated as an illness of society so they can control a higher percentage of the masses. In the case of health insurance, THEY created the problem ("addiction is a disease") and THEY provide the solution (they will vote to force insurance companies to pay for the treatment of addicts). I am not judging addicts, just stating how things occur.

Many physicians develop your treatment plan using the notion that, "If one patient had a bad experience due to this condition, then I must assume ALL patients will have a bad experience due to this."

To put it in other terms, Dr. Malcolm Kendrick brilliantly wrote: "Not all people who jump out of a plane without a parachute will die. But physicians treat us as if we will". He also states, as does Peggy Orenstein, author of *Our Feel-Good War on Breast Cancer*, that we must be able to look at our bodies as something that is good, and not as something that is due to kill us unless you go to a physician and seek all that can be sought.

Another example is that not ALL patients die from contracting the measles, but because "some" did, we are all forced to be vaccinated against this. Our politicians tell us it is for the good of the country, and perhaps they are correct, but they continue to place ALL illnesses into this category. (The truth is, measles are a potentially dangerous disease, so we should vaccinate enough people, 90 to 95% for a contagious disease such as measles, 80 to 85% for something less contagious like polio, in order for the "herd" to be protected; the vaccinated members of the herd do not transmit the disease to the unvaccinated.)

Again, it is so that they can control us and give us a reason to vote for them, and it makes money for the drug companies who support them, and the physicians who also donate to their candidacy.

Don't get me wrong; when our government is tasked with a crisis, it has done excellent work and performed miracles. World War I, World War II, The Marshall Plan and the rebuilding of Europe and Japan, NASA and the moon shot, the Internet, the Panama Canal, and the Manhattan Project are a few examples of our government taking on a monumental task and, by exerting a Herculean effort, they improved the lives of millions of people, here and abroad. But when it comes to the day-to-day task of running the country, most politicians are too busy focusing on getting re-elected to bother to make sure that the country is being run efficiently, and offtimes when they attempt to manage a perceived "crisis", it just winds up as another attempt to create a nanny state, with disastrous results with things like prohibition, and ridiculous regulations with the likes of banning smoking in bars and bans on large size servings of soft drinks, and flawed policies that led the US to have the highest rate of incarceration of any country in the world, with laws that severely penalize black people living in the US. The founding fathers stated in the Preamble of the Constitution that the role of government was to ensure that justice was served, and would protect its citizens from internal strife and from attack from the outside, and that it would be of benefit to the people, not a detriment, today and for future generations of Americans. The U.S. homicide rate is seven times that of other high-income countries, the second highest poverty rate, the highest obesity rate, the fewest hospital beds, the lowest life expectancy, the lowest rates of numeracy, the worst transportation infrastructure, the second highest deaths from car accidents, and the highest income inequality, all leading to the lowest voter turnout!

This equates to a grade of D- or F.

We Are All Born with an Expiration Date

(We are all going to die)

Stay with me on this one as I attempt to explain how organizations with agendas can influence others to go along for the ride.

I think about how the statement "we are all going to die" can silence most physicians and insurance companies, even politicians.

If you were to recommend your lawn care company to a neighbor, and the company gave you $20 off your next month's bill, would that not give you an incentive to recommend that company to another neighbor? I think it would, and it would be harmless.

What if I recommended a specialist dentist to you even though they were not the best that I was aware of, and they in turn recommended me to one of their patients? Is that harmless?

What if a government run insurance company reimburses physicians $25 to rehabilitate an injury, but paid $5,000 to perform surgery on that injury instead? Is that harmless? And which treatment do you think the physician would recommend?

And what if you go to your family physician for medication for a chronic condition, and they tell you that you must see a specialist for that medication? Is that correct? They justify it by thinking that the patient might sue them in 20 years for prescribing the medicine, yet their condition worsened. They are also influenced by an unspoken agreement with the specialist when they refer a patient and the specialist in turn refers patients back to the family practitioner. Is that harmless? Your insurance company reimburses the family physician only $25 to prescribe you something, but the specialist will be reimbursed $200 for a consultation and prescription.

In the mid-1900's, unions started to offer their members medical insurance. Physicians did not want to have to deal with paper work, phone calls to check insurance coverage, etc. The unions countered this resistance by selling a deal that encouraged patients to go to their physician or dentist every 6 months for exams, blood tests, tooth cleaning, etc.

The problem is this; the medical industrial complex and big government has taken a simple concept like health, the state of being free from illness or injury, and convinced us that all human beings are entitled to be "healthy." This is complete and utter nonsense! Some of us are born with bad genetics and are doomed to die long before the average human. Some of us will participate in risky behavior that will send us into a state of illness and/or injury and shorten our stay on the Earth. Others will be in the wrong place at the wrong time, due to life circumstances (like being born in an unstable country) or bad luck (like being hit by the Lite Beer truck). It is foolish to pursue such a policy.

The U.S. Government made a similar statement in the late 90's regarding home ownership, with some members of the House of Representatives stating that all Americans are entitled to own a home. Two presidents (Bill Clinton and George W. Bush) increased the quota of loans that Fannie Mae and Freddie Mac (the U.S. government's run mortgage company) made to people below the national medium income from 30 to 50% (Clinton, 2000), then to 55% (Bush, 2007). This prompted banks to develop sub-prime mortgage instruments (loans for buyers that are high risk), only to dump them on other banks that combined them with good loans, creating credit-default swaps, lowering the risk to investors. This all lead an instantaneous increase in the demand for housing, driving home prices up to unstainable levels. Existing homeowners took advantage of the increase in their home equity, borrowing against their homes and buying more "stuff", often with low initial interest rates which would only last a few years. Then in 2008, new and existing home owners were in a world of hurt as their mortgage payments increased and their home values plummeted to levels closer to the late 90's, and the value of credit-default swaps plummeted, causing a panic, resulting in the Great Recession. Not only did our government create the conditions to cause the Great Recession, they did nothing to punish the corrupt Wall Street bankers that made fortunes from exploiting the situation.

The Affordable Care Act has already created an imbalance in the demand and supply of healthcare, driving up costs at even faster rates than they had been rising. Once again, big government, now partnered with the Medical Industrial Complex, has the potential to create another unstainable situation. If they were to institute a single payer system (like Medicare for All) overnight, the disruption caused by the massive loss of jobs in the insurance industry would send the economy into another great recession instantly. And don't bet on them *not* doing something this catastrophic!

A perfect example of government sticking their nose in the wrong place and mucking everything up involves breast cancer. The ACA forced physicians to code the discovery of any tumor, benign or malignant, to be classified as "cancer." This allowed big government to present data to the public demonstrating that because of their "preventive" health insurance, there was an increase in identifying breast cancer, and to take credit for identifying life threatening conditions and saving lives. (And insuring that a major voting population (women) would keep voting for the Democratic Party, the folks that made the ACA possible!)

The simple truth is this; we are all born with an expiration date. There are lots of behaviors that can drastically reduce that date (risky behavior, consumption of toxic substances, abusing your body). Modern medicine has had advances, mostly around germ therapy that combatted infections (anti-biotics) and diseases that regularly wiped out large numbers of humans (vaccines), and technologies to detect disease (MRI) that have claimed increased longevity for a large number of humans that were not making it to their expected expiration dates. But at the end of the day, your genetics play a much more significant role then behavior.

Note: most studies put overall genetics as contributing 25 to 30% to your "expiration date." But they ignore two factors. First, your genetics play a major role in eight of the top ten causes of death (heart disease, cancer, chronic lower respiratory disease, stroke, Alzheimer's, diabetes, influenza and pneumonia, and kidney disease; only accidental death and suicide don't have a major genetic variation that we know for certain, but, are likely influenced by inherited behaviors). Second, inherited behavioral traits no doubt also lead to abusive behaviors that contribute to these behaviors (drug abuse, excessive smoking and drinking, to name just a few).

I studied evolution in great depth. All animals were selected through natural selection and luck, to continue in their genetic pool's life, if they lived to reproductive age, and then protected their kin long enough for them to reproduce. This means humans only have to live to 24 years in order for our species to avoid extinction, since females can reproduce at age 12; they then must only live to 24, or until their offspring can reproduce, again, at age 12.

So any life we experience after age 24 is simple luck or chance. Yet physicians act as if you must be treated in an attempt to live to 120 years, stating that is our biological age, and that if we do not live to that age, we have sinned and we have failed ourselves.

The Fallacy of Preventative Maintenance Exams (You must go to your physician regularly so we can find cancer before it kills you so that you can live forever)

Conspiracies are not necessarily planned actions. Sometimes they just occur and then others become co-conspirators by not protesting the actions taken by the conspirators.

The primary reason people go to the doctor every 6 or 12 months is because they think a doctor must tell them they found cancer or some other malady before the patient or another doctor discovers it. In doing so, the physicians can feel like a hero, and the patient can think that they did the right thing.

In reality, you have used most of your emotional capitol, your monetary capitol, and your time capitol (which could have better been spent with your friends and family), participating in a mirage.

We all will die of something. I say we all die from time. We cannot escape it. Everything in the universe sadly has a beginning and an end (Gribben, *In The Beginning*), but we must accept this and decide how we want to spend our time.

In *god is not Great*, Christopher Hitchens writes that religion exists to fill the need for our fear of death. Now the medical industrial complex is taking that need over from religions.

Instead of humans praying to a god, they pray to the medical industrial complex, hoping that, if they follow their physician's rules, or the latest health fad, they can avoid death.

Insurance Companies

You apply for life insurance in order to feel more secure, knowing that if you die prematurely, your children will get a head start in life. You call an insurance broker, and a nurse arrives at your door. The nurse says not to worry, they're just going to take your blood pressure and draw some blood to check your cholesterol level.

You are initially quoted $25 a month for the policy.

Two weeks later, you receive a letter with your new quote; $125 a month, with the explanation that you have high blood pressure and high cholesterol.

WTF?

This is how insurance companies and physicians conspire to pull the wool over our eyes, allowing both groups to make more money.

The insurance companies are there to make money, not to give you an honest deal. They create excuses to charge you more, saying you are likely to die sooner if you have high blood pressure or high cholesterol readings.

Physicians check you for both of these as most patients are likely to go along with the scam and accept the tests, being afraid to look foolish by asking why, and where is the evidence? The media has convinced them/us that these are legitimate problems.

There is no evidence that blood pressure or cholesterol effects how long we live. To the contrary, there are well carried out research projects that demonstrate the exact opposite, that blood pressure and cholesterol levels have no effect on longevity.

The Sell

"Ask your doctor if you have low T"

When did all the abbreviations start? Why?

I remember the first medical abbreviations had to do with things that embarrassed patients, so physicians thought if the patients don't have to say the actual words, maybe they will not be afraid to ask for the service.

A perfect example of this is ED (erectile dysfunction) for men who desire a better sex life. Most cases were due to low testosterone. Testosterone received a bad rap when it was linked to athletes using it as a performance enhancing drug (which is in doubt). So the medical community started using the term "Low T", thinking this would free shy men from talking about their problem. I don't know if it worked, but now almost all medical conditions are abbreviated on TV for the purposes of encouraging patients into asking for treatment and examination of ailments, and we are inundated with pitches for products to help men with ED.

The new and "improved" examination for blood sugar is now referred to as "A1C". Low testosterone is "Low T". And there are many others you will notice if you watch even a few hours of TV or listen to the radio.

STD's replace all variety of embarrassing maladies caused by unprotected sex, UTI's describe any difficulty you're having peeing, and absorbent products replaces adult diapers. Doctors have their own jargon for talking bad about their customers (us)! A surgeon operating on someone with HIV will use the term "High Five", a "code brown" is a patient with diarrhea, a child with a genetic or congenital condition affecting their appearance becomes a FLK, or Funny Looking Kid, people that are overusing the ER for non-emergencies are referred to as "frequent flyers", OB-GYN's talk about "harpooning the whale" when they have to insert an epidural catheter to provide pain meds and, worse of all, patients that die are "discharged up", as in, discharged to heaven!

This expansion of our medical vocabulary by either using abbreviations or by inundating us with advertisements for drugs that will cure a "problem" that they are convincing us that we have is now a major part of most American's life. It feels like more people have stronger brand loyalty about choosing between Advil versus Motrin, Crest White Strips versus Rembrandt Whitening Strips, and Xanax versus Valium, over choosing between the Yankees versus the Mets, or their favorite brand of automobile!

GOOD SCIENCE:
THE MALAY ARCIPELAGO
VOLUMES 1 AND 2

I decided to dedicate an entire section to Alfred Russel Wallace, author of the *Malay Archipelago, Volumes 1 and 2.*

Alfred Russel Wallace was born in 1823. He did not have access to information as we now have at our disposal 24/7. He did not have a telephone, television, cell phone, or computer. He did not have access to the internet. Even publications were a rare thing in his day.

In 1869, Wallace published one of the greatest recordings of nature ever made, *The Malay Archipelago.* Prior to this, he had made journeys to the Amazon rain forest in South America.

His transportation was in a wooden ship, both to the Amazon and Malaysia. No refrigeration or air conditioning. He was not able to call home if he wanted to know how to describe a life form he encountered. All he had was the information in his head from years of observation and studying in England. He did not graduate high school, nor did he attend a university. He was a naturalist who studied all living things.

He described thousands of new species of plants and animals, described in detail ocean currents and climates without access to satellite photos or outside information. He accurately described the islands of Malaysia and answered why the fauna and flora was the same or different on each island. He independently conceived the theory of evolution through natural selection when Darwin was writing *On the Origin of the Species.*

How did he accomplish this?

How? How? How?

Was he from another planet? Was he a super human?

No. He was a scientist who studied in the correct manner and was not afraid to state his findings, even if someone else did not agree with him.

He was the first real bio-geologist.

I believe that Alfred Russel Wallace was what ALL physicians and dentists should be expected to be. He flew by the seat of his pants. He made an observation and described what it was, and was able to draw from previous works to come up with an explanation or description of what he experienced.

Nowadays, a similarly eager explorer would not bother to study as much as Wallace. Instead, they would be sure to take plenty of batteries with them and would be scanning images of what they saw and sending them electronically to a colleague who had access to encyclopedias, most likely on the internet.

Since he did not have knowledge of what came before him, he would most likely be guilty of plagiarizing many authors. But who would care?

Modern physicians and dentists should prepare themselves for an adventure as great as that of Wallace prior to practicing medicine or dentistry, but they do not.

Modern physicians and dentists don't know what is normal. Wallace could look at the skeletal remains of a rare vertebrate and know within a centimeter if it was in the limits of a male or female, or if it was an anomalous size. Modern physicians and dentists would order an expensive set of unnecessary X-rays or DNA lab tests, then read the lab results that would tell them what diagnosis to make. Modern physicians and dentists cannot tell what is in the normal by simple observation and are afraid to try techniques due to fear of being sued if they were wrong.

I urge all physicians and dentists to read the *Malay Archipelago* so that they can understand how a real scientist practices science and to understand what they should be doing, so they can be sure of what they know and to trust that they are correct no matter what social media tells them, and, so that will not allow consensus to guide them.

Wallace prepared himself for a great adventure. Doctors and dentists should prepare themselves in a similar manner as Wallace did for practicing medicine and dentistry.

I observed the following; a 25 year-old man is at a popular children's park on a hot, humid day. He looks pale, and says he feels weak. What should be done?

A physician who has the proper background and mindset should lie him down, place ice around his head, give him liquids, and wait for him to recover.

What happens in our current world where healthcare has gone wild? The physician on call first thinks, "What must I do to not be sued? Is there a one percent chance this guy might die? Maybe he has cancer, or a heart condition. I should order a CT scan prior to treating him, and an EKG to rule out a heart attack. I need to be safe (translation, avoid a lawsuit)."

So a simple case of heat stroke turns into a ruined day for the tourist as he is billed for an ambulance ride, CT scan and EKG, and IV liquids after passing out from a simple case of heat stroke. All because physicians first think about themselves and law suits. Instead of addressing the patient's problem and allowing him to return to a fun day, he is made into an emergency patient due to a physician's fear of a lawsuit and his reputation.

Consider another example; you have diarrhea. You need some simple Over-the-Counter medicine to hold you over. But your Internist insists you get a colonoscopy and endoscopy before they will diagnose and treat you.

Just because something can be done doesn't mean it should be done. But, of course, they will justify it by telling themselves that they are avoiding a future law suit, and the extra tests will make their practice a lot of money.

As stated earlier, there is an increase in drowning deaths when people consume more ice cream. Correlation does not imply causation. But physicians treat us all as if we will all if we eat ice cream and go swimming.

Another example; I have ulcerative colitis. It can be diagnosed by a simple X-ray and symptoms. My physician insists on performing a colonoscopy to look for inflammatory cells in my large intestine. It was not needed. It can be done, but is not needed (just because it can be done does not mean it should be done). Next, I was put on corticosteroids and antibiotics to treat a fever.

For years, I continued to suffer from periodic flare-ups. I found a doctor (not a specialist) who gave me some medicine which helped me greatly, but still did not stop my hiccups and gastric reflux from a hiatal hernia. My gastro intestinal specialist told me to go to the emergency room every time I suffered from a flare-up. I asked how am I supposed to lead a normal life not knowing when a flare-up will occur, and then having to go to the ER. My physician merely shrugs his shoulders and avoided answering my question. As a scientist, I decided to conduct my own research with the goal of discovering a better way to treat my condition, and not trust the so-called "specialists." My research (which included reading numerous research papers and participating in chat rooms on the internet) gave me information on what to expect with my illness.

So it appears that my so called "specialist" was more interested in performing a colonoscopy on me than in giving me a good quality of life. And he assumed that my quality of life was insignificant, that I lived to serve "him".

Analogy; you have a car and the tire is flat from a slow leak. Alfred Russel Wallace would put a patch on the tire, fill the tire with air, and send you on your way.

What would today's physicians do? They would check the tire's air pressure and document that the tire needed air, then check the other tires and balance all of the wheels to determine if that gave them any information they could use to diagnose the problem. They would then put air in the flat tire and send you on your way. You ask why they didn't patch the hole, and are told that if it runs out of air again, have it towed in, and they will put air in it again, as they fear being sued if their repair job failed.

This is what our healthcare system has come to. The physician's goal is not to heal you or to make your life better. Rather, it is to perform expensive, unnecessary procedures on you and then leave you in a situation of fear and insecurity. What seems to matter most to patients (getting out of a painful short term condition) tends to be ignored by the physicians and dentists.

Another way to think of the medical industrial complex is as a sophisticated virus. A successful virus is a small parasite that cannot reproduce itself; it requires a host, and a method to be inserted initially into the host, and another method to spread. Viruses are also known to mutate, making them harder to destroy. Some viruses kill the host before spreading, thus ending their existence. But a "smart" virus enters the host, mutates, then just draws enough out of the host to live and thrive without killing the host.

In this example, the medical industrial complex is the virus, and you are the host. The virus is introduced to the host at birth, first by an OB-GYN, then a pediatrician, then a family practitioner. In order for the virus to make an impact, it needs to get the host, you, on meds, either by prescribing them, or sending you to a specialist to prescribe them. Once you start these meds, it's hard to stop. Most people stay on blood pressure and cholesterol meds for life once they start them. But that's not enough. Because the meds often have side effects, the host receives additional meds to combat the impact of the side effects. This is the mutation process. Before you know it, you are taking a dozen different meds every day.

The medical industrial complex can keep you alive, slowly draining you of life and of your bank account, for a very long time.

What a sophisticated virus!

To quote from the TV series *Seinfeld* in the episode *The Heart Attack*, "The medical establishment is a business like any other business. And business needs customers. And, they want to sell you their most expensive item which is unnecessary surgery. You see, it's in the best interest of the medical profession that you remain sick. You see, that insures good business. You're not a patient. You're a customer."

PROBLEMS

MYTHS/FADS

Myths: Everything and nothing

As I stated in the Foundations chapter, the medical and dental profession are void of test pilots. The wise men who carried out true research, who asked the right questions and assumed nothing, who presented their findings no matter what the outcome, no longer exist.

Now it is more important that a physician be famous or that he get attention from a social group he might be a member of.

How myths are started is most likely due to human nature. Even now, we can see animals teaching their young what to eat. Different species (lions, birds, apes) learn what is safe to eat by observing their parents. If a parent were to eat a deadly plant or animal and its children copied this behavior, their genetic material would not be passed on as they would have died before reaching reproductive age.

This behavior also exists in humans. Most back pains will pass in time. If you were eating grapes at the time the back pain ceased, you most likely would attribute this alleviation of pain to a diet of grapes, you would then instruct your children of the value of grapes, and this behavior would be passed on.

Myths in diet are probably the largest category of myths related to healthcare. They have greatly infiltrated our healthcare system, with physicians and dentists both instructing their patients on what to consume with no research as evidence. They simply "believe" it to be true.

Most of us have now been "mythed" into thinking that we must pay attention to the word "nutrient." All living things have nutrients in them. But your advisors want you to think that "they" know what "nutrients" are best for you, or which foods have the best "nutrients."

The blood pressure myth has been passed on from generation to generation, along with the cholesterol myth.

It is scientifically known that what we eat does not affect longevity. Most of us incorrectly believe that the Japanese eat only plants, and no carbohydrates. Recently, researchers have gone back to these towns in Japan where these myths were started and it was found that these long living people were actually eating 90% carbohydrates. Will this finding make it into this week's headlines? I seriously doubt it, since the editors will not want to publish something that goes against their beliefs.

Cancer and high blood pressure; an example

First of all, there is no such thing as high blood pressure. But if I were to ask, "What causes cancer or high blood pressure", I would have to say, "Everything and nothing."

And I say the above because these assumptions are made on the basis of non-research. What the "experts" mistook for research were actually essays of surveys which did not include only one variable and which were not based on direct observation, but instead, were based on surveys which can be manipulated by persons with agendas, or by persons who do not know what research is.

A very extensive study was carried out in the 1970's in an attempt to find out if warming up and stretching prevented athletic injuries. This same research was once again carried out in the 2000's. Both researchers came up with the same data and conclusions: stretching and warming up did nothing to prevent injuries. These actions of stretching and warming up only served as "rituals" for teams to form a sense of "sameness" among its team mates. The same with blood pressure. It is a ritual and is not backed by any science.

Cancer is primarily the result of bad luck involving either genetics, viruses or chemicals. Most cells in your body are periodically making copies of themselves. In rare instances, they make a random mistake (mutation) which can possibly lead to cancer and accelerate the time period when the copies are being made (causing the cancer to metastasize).

Some studies produced good evidence that cancers are primarily caused by viruses. This came about when they studied what cancer occurred where and at what time. It was discovered that different cancers seemed to travel in waves around the globe in much the same way as infectious viruses.

Radiation does not cause cancer, although some forms can cause damage to living organisms. Pundits of radiation causing cancer surprisingly make references to studies from the Hiroshima and Nagasaki nuclear bombs of WWII, but they use the information incorrectly. Independent studies AND studies from government funded associations BOTH state that populations exposed to nuclear radiation have LESS cases of cancer.

The sad truth is, the longer we live, the greater the chance for these triggers to cause genetic mistakes in our cells. If and when science finds a way to get humans to regularly live into their hundreds, we will all eventually contract cancer. The same is true for wild animals kept in zoos. In the wild, a slight malfunction in physical ability (fitness) equals death from predators, or the inability of a predator to catch prey. In zoos, where predators are kept at bay, the animals live longer and die of cancer.

Fads: when fads become trends

"Religions were created by humans because they were afraid of death." (Hitchens, *god is not Great*).

It is part of human nature to fear death (for most of us). Our medical industrial complex has hijacked this desire to protect ourselves from death. We can be "fooled" by snake oil salesmen with their promise of "magic" potions and "nutrients". Every month a new plant is sold as the next great snake oil, and many of us fall for this.

Think germs are bad? Think you can rid your body of them? 10 years ago, a medical student calculated that there are more bacterial cells in the human body than human cells. Numerous scientific groups have studied the role of bacteria in our body and conclude that the ratio is about 1:1.

Bacteria are everywhere and we cannot make ourselves safer by killing them all. We need them to live. Hand sanitizers kill our natural bacteria, those that protects us from foreign, harmful bacteria, and then, the sanitizers pollute our rivers and water supplies.

The above are all fads. Stories that appear in some form of media about things that people use or do that get your friends all worked up are excellent sources for fads. Fads exist because we want to do what everyone else is doing, or because we think we are being smart in discovering some "secret" solution.

Myths and Fads: The List

You must get all of the following myths and fads out of your head if you are to advance yourself to being able to live in the reality of your choice.

1. You can prevent death from **cancer** if you go to regular medical exams and have your physician screen for cancer; colon, prostate and breast cancer can be beaten if you find them early
2. Blood thinners are required to prevent **stroke and heart attacks**
3. **Blood pressure** matters
4. **Cholesterol** matters
5. **Irritable bowel syndrome** flare ups can be prevented
6. You have to take **vitamins** to get your nutritional needs met and this benefits you.
7. A **balanced diet** is a scientific term that you must achieve and fad diets benefit your health
8. **Exercise** prolongs life
9. You have to ingest **probiotics** to correct your gut flora
10. Make sure you take those **antibiotics** your doctor prescribes to stay healthy
11. **Diabetes** is treatable with insulin and treatment leads to a longer life; diabetes is incurable
12. Name brand **drugs** are superior to generics
13. We should do whatever we can to extend life when you're on your death bed (**palliative care**)
14. If we don't need a **body part** or it might become cancerous someday, just cut it out
15. Chiropractors, Homeopathy and Acupuncture (**alternative medicine**) work

16. **Dental matters**; you have to brush, floss and get your teeth cleaned regularly if you want to keep them
17. Systemic **fluoride** is bad
18. **Periodontal disease** (gum disease) is caused by local irritants in your gums
19. Your **silver fillings** can kill you
20. **Dental X-rays** cause cancer
21. Your shrink is giving you the best advice…and meds (**mental health**)
22. **Stress** is bad
23. We must go to medical **specialists** to treat everything
24. You can control whether or not you **live to be 100**

Cancer

Question: What are the causes of cancer?

Answer: Everything and nothing. So don't sweat it.

What does that word do to you? Does it make you sweat? That is what the medical industrial complex wants it to do to you.

First, think about this. Can you think of any food or man-made object that has NOT been labeled as causing cancer by someone or some institution?

You must think a long time. Has water consumption ever been linked to cancer? The answer is yes! Even water has been accused of causing cancer if it is bottled in certain containers.

Radiation has NEVER been observed to cause cancer. The sun has never been shown to cause cancer. The nuclear bombs dropped on Japan have never resulted in a single case of cancer. But every one of you reading this book has been taught that these were irrefutable truths.

The four major causes of all cancers are, in order:

1. Genetics
2. Viruses
3. Chemicals
4. Time

I hope you noticed that radiation and sunshine are not on the list.

What happened to all the ads about using sunscreen in order to prevent skin cancer? The sun does not cause cancer. Melanoma has occurred in many places where the sun doesn't shine. How can this be? The physicians on TV tell you that you will die if you go in the sun. Why was this not a problem in past centuries? The media has an answer for this; we have changed our climate so we now have a greater probability of getting skin cancer. They have an answer for everything, as they know much about what is not. (Ronald Reagan).

Simply put, radiation does not cause cancer; experimentation has shown that natural genetic mutations occur at a higher rate than radiation related genetic mutations. Therefore, any genetic change that radiation causes is overshadowed by natural biology.

Big government has the answer, they can solve all of our problems! Good thing; they often are the cause of many of them!

These myths come and go at the convenience of politicians. Big government wants all of the population to think that only government can save you. So big government creates big problems, then present the solutions, which is more big government.

Unfortunately, most of us will be convinced to have many unnecessary medical procedures performed on our bodies because we have been brainwashed into thinking that we are a mechanical Mr. Potato Head. Every day you hear a co-worker say that it's time to have their car's oil changed, or get a 50,000 mile check-up. This instills auto plausibility in us. We think our car will last forever if we change the oil regularly and that if something fails it was our fault for not having it checked regularly. Evidence does not support this. But it makes sense to us. It seems plausible.

The fact is, all mechanical parts will eventually fail. In truth, EVERYTHING in the universe eventually comes to an end (*Understanding Why, evolution, beliefs and your reality*).

The great science fiction author Isaac Asimov observed, "If entropy must constantly and continuously increase, then the universe is remorselessly running down, thus setting a limit on the existence of humanity."

Is Cancer Curable?

A famous British journalist in the late 1990's/early 2000's was diagnosed and treated for breast cancer. She submitted to surgery, radiation and chemo treatments. She did what the specialists told her would cure her, and was told that she would live forever. 10 years after completing treatment, she was diagnosed with untreatable and terminal breast cancer. She was furious. Why did she suffer through the emotional pain of surgery and then the physical illness brought on by the radiation and chemo treatments if she was going to die anyway?

Peggy Orenstein chronicled a similar story in *Our Feel-Good War on Breast Cancer.* (More on that shorty).

A "search for the cure" is pure fantasy.

Physicians in medical schools continue to battle one another on the definition of "cure". To some it means the complete absence of any of the cancer that you were being treated for.

To others it means you live for 5 years after the treatment is "complete" for that cancer. Yet to others it means you died of time from something else, not the cancer you were treated for.

The first journalist in this story was on a mission to find the truth about breast cancer, and to understand why her doctors were ignorant, and why they misinformed her.

She used her journalist credentials to travel the world and attend as many breast cancer lectures as she could. She concluded that breast cancer only had two forms. One killed you no matter what treatment you underwent. The other did not kill you no matter what treatment you had done. So there is no value in having mammograms, mastectomies, chemo or radiation therapy; all of those treatments do not effect what will happen to you. But they will rob you of your financial and emotional capitol and take you away from your loved ones, and from experiencing the joy of life.

A pair of papers published in 2017 backed up the previously mentioned journalist's conclusions by stating that no cancers can be cured and that specifically, breast cancer prevention does not exist. Genetic screening means nothing and treatments do not affect your outcome.

Breast cancer? Why did the propaganda change from, "'A Race for the Cure" to "Breast Cancer Awareness"?

Searching for cancer in an attempt to live a normal and long life is simply mental masturbation.

Some of us are born to be 4 feet tall, some 8 feet tall. Some of us will be geniuses, some idiots. Some will grow cancer and die of it, some will grow cancer and live a "normal" life.

We all live with the cards we are dealt.

Our medical institutions and politicians want us to think we can change our destiny with cancer, and that we should "fight it". According to some politicians who are always looking for a reason to seek our vote in perpetuity, it is our "right" to fight it.

In contrast, Orenstein wrote "we must stop making women think that their breasts, ovaries and cervix are time bombs, waiting to go off."

Government thinks if they connect an emotional reaction to a cause, you will donate all your money to them. That is how the phrase "fight for the cause" was created. If your child had cancer, they only died because YOU didn't fight hard enough.

Having a painful death or fatal illness can happen to anyone. It is a consequence of being alive. Most of us think that we must look for it and have it treated. This decision will rob you of your financial and emotional capitol, leaving you with a wasted life.

Virtually NO cancer screening has been shown to reduce cancer deaths OR to prolong a person's life. Yet all physicians and many dentists continue to perform these screening exams, charging the patient for them. Their reasoning; it is politically correct (not to mention financially profitable for the medical industrial complex). Patients receive these exams at other offices and will think you are not giving them everything you should since other physicians or dentists are doing it.

If you discover that you have cancer and your physician did not screen you for it, you might decide to sue them. And as mentioned previously, there is an oversupply of lawyers in the U.S. to satisfy our litigious minded, dissatisfied medical industrial complex customers. This only serves to drive malpractice insurance rates up, which in turn drive up healthcare costs.

Our medical schools must do a better job of differentiating from real research and political correctness.

Are you embarrassed?

Breast cancer. Prostate cancer. Colon cancer. Oddly, all deal with our "private" areas. Seems that when something concerns our loved ones privates, we are suckers to leave all logic behind and go into poverty in order to help "cure" them. We believe all the fads, all the commercials.

Facts are, these cancers, when studied properly, are found to not be susceptible to preventive or curative methods.

Dr. Richard Ablin, the man who discovered the PSA (prostate specific antigen, which is now a blood test that is incorrectly used to detect prostate cancer), told the audience in a 2015 radio interview about his search for information to validate that his PSA test did not indeed prevent unnecessary prostate cancer deaths.

The PSA was identified by Ablin to give a physician a statistical measure of the probability of a patient's prostate cancer returning after having had prostate cancer treatment. The blood test, invented by a pharmaceutical company, cannot and was never meant to determine if a patient had a cancerous prostate.

Ablin decided to investigate what physicians used to determine if a patient had prostate cancer. In doing so, Ablin asked colleagues who treated prostate cancer, what research they referred to which, in their minds, validated that prostate exams helped patients. They first referred him to a paper on the PSA test. He contacted the author of the paper and asked where his research was stored and for permission to examine his data. The author flat out refused. In classical research terms, this invalidates anything in the published results. If a scientist askes to view your data and specimens and you cannot produce either, it raises a big red flag on your work.

Ablin approached his colleagues again and told them of his experience and observation, and that the paper was a fake. Again he asked them what they based their practices on. They presented another paper to him. Once again, he contacted the author who seemed to be very nervous as Ablin explained to him who he was, and that he wanted to examine the research material.

Not only did the author refuse to allow him to examine his materials, but he broke down and admitted that he did not perform any actual research, that, in fact, he combined other studies, added each publication's number of patients together, and claimed that he had examined all of these patients.

Ablin now states that no physician under any circumstance should screen men for prostate cancer using any means until proper research is conducted to find if any testing is useful in prostate screening. Basically, any prostate screening is pure "snake oil"!

A recent article published in the BBC stated that there is no test to detect prostate cancer.

Medicaid and the VA (in decisions made by politicians), decided to offer the PSA test to its patients as a benefit, even though it was not intended to find prostate cancer. As a result, other medical insurances followed this ignorant decision. And now your husbands and sons are undergoing unnecessary prostate surgeries and experiencing quality of life vacuums.

How many men have had their lives destroyed by having a death sentence given to them by an ignorant physician? How many had to wear diapers for the remaining precious years of their life, or not been able to have sex, all as a result of unnecessary surgery?

What about colon cancer? We are told that we must get a regular checkup every year starting at age 40. Sound familiar? We all have automobiles and are told we must have the oil changed every 3,000 miles. The mechanic even places a sticker in front of your face to remind you of how important it is. It is mechanic plausible. We easily adapt that to the bio plausible logic and conclude that we must have regular checkups in order to live a long life. The problem is, research in the past decades has proven that automobiles that did not have oil changes in their first 100,000 miles did not have any more "preventable" problems occurring to them than those that had regular oil changes. But it is mechanical plausible, so we do it and do not question our actions.

Colonoscopies have not been shown to benefit a patient in a preventive manner. If you are experiencing intestinal problems, a colonoscopy can help identify the problem, but simple abdominal X-rays and lab tests can be used to diagnose the problem. Arbitrarily performing colonoscopies on patients only serves to fill the physician and hospital's bank accounts, and these invasive exams can lead to life threatening injuries that are unnecessary.

If polyps are identified and removed, the process does not lessen a patient's chance of coming down with colon cancer.

In fact, a recent literature review of ulcerative colitis (UC) articles found that 50% of the articles found a higher rate of colon cancer among UC patients; the other 50% showed NO difference in the incidence of colon cancer among UC sufferers. And even the articles that claim an association of colon cancer to patients with UC, they only claim a 3% association.

So, looking at the entire picture, if there is any association between colon cancer and UC, it is close to zero. But your physician will attempt to scare the bejeebers out of you and scare you into agreeing to stool tests, colonoscopies and biopsies.

Chemotherapy has been getting a healthy dose of criticism lately, but not nearly enough in my mind. The whole idea behind chemotherapy is this; chemotherapy has come to connote non-specific usage of intracellular poisons to inhibit mitosis (cell division). In layman's terms, it is a poison designed to attack cells that reproduce quickly (cancer cells, but also hair follicles, cells in the mouth, digestive tract and reproductive organs, and bone marrow) with the hopes of killing the fast growing cells while only temporarily damaging the rest of the body. It is a process that slowly kills you as it seeks out your cancer. Sounds like bloodletting, a practice that had a 2,500 year run, and leach therapy, which is still used! A recent study concluded that chemotherapy only improves the five-year survival rate by 2 percentage points.

A recent study on breast cancer found that chemotherapy most likely did not help anyone. All of these woman had their breasts removed, followed by losing their hair. And for what? A theory?

Other studies indicate that chemotherapy actually causes damage long after the treatment is completed. The more common side effects include early menopause and weight gain. Less common side effects include hearing loss, heart problems, infertility, nerve damage, osteoporosis, reduced lung capacity, loss of taste and, last and but not least, increased risks of other cancers. Another recent study determined that chemotherapy administered before surgery (called neoadjuvant chemotherapy) might actually promote the spread of other cancers.

If you had a cancer that kills you no matter what, you are scalded by your physician and family, and are told that you did not get tested early enough, or frequently enough, or that you ate the wrong foods, or that you smoked too much, or that you drank too much alcohol. You are blamed for your short, bad life by ignorant people who are very misinformed. You want to do the "right" thing, as you perceive your friends do, in order to avoid social "shame" from your peers.

In *Our Feel-Good War on Breast Cancer*, Peggy Orenstein is very adamant that searching for breast cancer does not benefit the patient at all. That this "war" turns young woman into thinking that their sexual organs are time bombs, and this prevents them from enjoying the body they were born with, all due to political correctness, stupidity, and greed.

Bill was diagnosed with testicular cancer (embryonal carcinoma, the type that Lance Armstrong had) in 2002. The cancerous testis was removed (radical orchiectomy) and the cancer was determined to be stage one. He was given two options for post op treatment. The first and more commonly taken was to go into a five year period of remission and have abdominal CT scans every six months to search for the possibility that the cancer had metastasized and was in the abdominal lymph nodes. The second was to have three weeks of light abdominal radiation which would eradicate any undetectable cancer that had spread from the testis and be declared cured. Since this type of cancer is easily destroyed by radiation, he choose the radiation therapy, even though it was guaranteed to cause a loss of appetite, extreme nausea, and weight loss. But the factor that drove him to seek the more unpleasant treatment was the fact that he was allergic to iodine. CT scans with contrast required iodine injections. Even though the ingestion of a steroid 24 hours before the CT scan would almost certainly eliminate an allergic reaction to the iodine, he was not willing to take that chance ten times over the next five years; one defective steroid pill could lead to his going into anaphylactic shock, a condition that can result in death.

Vascular Diseases (strokes and heart attacks)

Blood thinners; the cure all? They are very bio plausible, but do they work? The long and short answer is "no"; they simply don't allow a clot to kill you. But they can create a new problem that kills you, "bleeding strokes".

Blood thinners are often prescribed to treat some types of heart disease and heart defects, as well as to "prevent" heart attacks and/or strokes. About 2 to 3 million Americans have prescriptions for blood thinners.

Many of the above observations have been also made by Dr. Malcolm Kendrick in a series of essays. He goes further by saying that something that causes disease or discomfort in one person does not mean it causes it in "ALL" people. But that is how the medical industrial complex behaves.

There are long lived people who claim to have smoked tobacco most of their lives, have eaten fried and barbequed food for most of their lives, who have not eaten "balanced" diets for most of their lives, and who have not exercised for most of their lives. Yet most of us will starve ourselves of those "quality of life" inducing charms, identified above, in the name of fads and myths that promise to keep us alive forever.

Yes, these people lived full lives. They enjoyed a full quality of life by consuming what they desired.

And the one other thing that they all had in common was that they did NOT participate in a medical industrial complex that is "improving" our lives.

Up until the 1960's, most people that had heart attacks in the developed world were sent home and told to adapt a sedentary life style, that their hearts were sick and that they should never again be put under undo stress, including sex. It wasn't until ground breaking work on aerobics was conducted by Dr. Kenneth Cooper, the man known as the father of aerobics (*Aerobics*, Kenneth Cooper, *1968*) showed that the heart, like any other muscle, needs to be conditioned and exercised, and that recovery from a heart attack should include exercise once the body is ready for it.

This, however, does not prolong life or reduce heart problems; it merely allows the person to return to an active life style, who was previously condemned to a sedentary one.

High Blood Pressure

We've already covered this topic pretty thoroughly. To summarize, HBP (high blood pressure) became a "problem" only after big pharma discovered a "solution". How can 50% of the world's adult population be classified with a condition (HBP)?

Cholesterol

Myth #1: Cholesterol is bad. Wrong! Cholesterol helps produce hormones, cell membranes and vitamin D, it aids in digestion, and it is important for cognitive function (it helps you to form memories).

Myth #2: There is such a thing as bad and good cholesterol. They are described thusly: Bad cholesterol (LDL) kills. Wrong! A recent study invalidated the hypothesis that high LDL cholesterol is the main cause of heart disease, "because people with low levels become just as atherosclerotic (hardened arteries) as people with high levels and their risk of suffering from CVD (Cardio Vascular Disease) is the same or higher." In fact, good cholesterol (HDL) might not be as "good" as we've been told. A new study published in *European Heart Journal* determined that HDL may raise the risk of premature death

Even the global medical industrial complex cannot agree on a definition for "high" cholesterol.

- USA: over 200 milligrams per deciliter of blood (212 mg/dL)
- UK: over 5 millimoles per liter (mmol/L) of blood (193 mg/dL)
- Canada: over 6.2 mmol/L (240 mg/dL)
- France: over 6.5 mmol/L (251 mg/dL)
- Japan doesn't bother much with cholesterol testing

Irritable Bowel Syndrome (IBS)

Physicians, when examining patients for IBS, will take a visual look with a colonoscopy, and take a sample of the mucus lining of the intestines. The physician then tells his patient that the inflammation caused his condition of bleeding diarrhea, then sends them running to the pharmacist or to their office to treat them with anti-inflammatory medicines, instructing them not to eat certain foods because they "think" that they increase inflammation in your body, and hence, in your intestines, and in doing so, will cure you of your debilitating condition.

The problem is, a highly respected medical school performed an extensive study of the literature and concluded that there is NOTHING a patient can do to prevent a flare-up of irritable bowel conditions. NOTHING.

So, then, why does your physician insist on changing your diet, medications, and mental health condition (they also will tell you that stress causes flare-ups)? The best answer is bio plausibility, along with ignorance. They simply listen to what other physicians have told them, rather than listen to patients who are suffering from the condition. They see inflammatory cells in the biopsy and assume that the inflammation must have caused the condition.

When a patient is on a cortisone medicine to "prevent" a flare-up, they are actually "treating" a flare-up that is not there. When one does occur, you already are taking the prescribed cure. So why take medicine for something you do not have? Would you take an ibuprofen each day because it prevents a headache? It would not be preventing anything; it would be treating you each day for a headache whether or not you have one.

I consulted with 5 physicians about my ulcerative colitis and if I played their responses one after the other most of us would be bent over while laughing at their ridiculous advice.

A balanced diet/nutrition/in moderation

Whole foods are defined as a food that one can eat and receive all the necessary ingredients an individual requires to live a normal, fit life. An example of a whole food is a bird egg or a chicken with the skin on.

So who decided what a "balanced" diet is anyway? (Balanced and in moderation are used in similar manners). During hard times, humans have survived by eating insects (80% of the planet currently consumes insects as a regular part of their diet). Some only had access to fruit, or carrion, or raw fish.

So WHO came up with this "balanced" diet idea?

The U.S. Department of Agriculture, that's who. USDA Dietary Guidelines were invented in order to keep the American people eating farm grown food in order to keep farmers employed. The USDA came up with the concept of a balanced diet in 1894, but it wasn't until 1992 when they created the food guide pyramid that the USDA went off the rails and really led the American public astray. The 1992 guideline initially emphasized eating more vegetables and fruits, less meat, salt, sugary foods, "bad" fats, and additive-rich factory foods (aka, "processed" foods). But the food industrial complex (farmers and food manufacturers) intervened, fearing lost sales, bought off their politicians, and the pyramid was changed. Over the 10+ years following the 1992 guidelines, obesity rates in the U.S. doubled; the guidelines not only encouraged the over consummation of grains (which are calorically dense and tend to be consumed in over refined states), vilified all fat consumption (including fats essential for proper body processes) and failed to define portion size. The result; obesity rates went from 15% in 1990 to 36% by 2012. A 2004 study in the *Journal of the American Physicians and Surgeons* determined that there was little doubt that there was "a clear temporal association between the 'heart healthy' diet and the current, growing epidemics of cardiovascular disease, obesity and Type 2 diabetes."

As stated earlier, some government agencies site a Japanese population's diet for their longevity. This population was recently studied once again to confirm that the earlier conclusion of the study were correct. It was found that the study group consumed a diet of 90% carbohydrates, which our government states is "bad" for us.

If there is such a thing as a "balanced" diet, what is balanced? What does "eating in moderation" mean? If we use the term balance in physics, it refers to two masses or forces on either side of a fulcrum, such as a see-saw, being equal.

I have never come across any scientific publication that examined what a balanced diet was. It is a nonsense term that has no use in diet or health, yet I have heard many physicians tell their patients to eat a balanced diet.

I hear colleagues at work saying they are eating "healthy", or that they are consuming a balanced diet. Who decides what the two foods are that are to be in "balance"? How did they arrive at these foods?

Who is the authority in deciding this?

Let me just say, ignore everything that you hear or read that has to do with a "balanced" diet. It does not exist, nor does a "healthy" diet.

There is no observed way of choosing what we eat that is beneficial to your longevity. Interestingly, babies, when presented with all of the food groups at every meal, will eventually, over the course of less than a week, select foods which will fill any deficiency in their body.

Vitamins

Linus Pauling was a famous scientist who won two Noble Prizes. In 1962, he went down a path of destruction. (The *Vitamin Myth: Why WE Think WE Need Supplements,* Paul Offit, July 19, 2013, *Atlantic*). Pauling started telling people that vitamin C was a miracle vitamin and that it cured colds, cancers and most other maladies. He had no evidence of this. He just went off on a dark adventure.

As Pauling was a famous Noble Prize winning scientist, people of course followed his recommendation and started taking vitamin C in large quantities. The age of supplemental vitamins had begun.

Over the years, many long term studies have demonstrated that taking daily vitamins shortens a human's life span.

Pauling and his wife both consumed large quantities of vitamin C every day and were sure it was the elixir of life.

In 1994, Pauling and his wife both died of cancer.

Did you take your vitamins today? Why? Did you ever research whether or not they help you?

Truth is, it is very difficult to become vitamin deficient. During WW2, some Europeans became deficient in vitamin C due to a lack of fresh fruit. Vitamin manufacturers took advantage of the situation and advertised that everyone needed vitamins, and that all you had to do was take their magic pills in order to get them.

Pauling added fuel to the fire.

Our obsession with anti-oxidants is the equivalent with our past obsession with vitamin C.

Exercise

Long term studies and observations demonstrate that people engaged in physically demanding jobs have an 18% greater risk of dying early. Some have fabricated a certain amount of exercise that is the optimal amount for mental and cardiovascular well-being. Our cells can only perform a finite amount of biochemical processes. The more we eat and exert, the faster we use up these finite amounts of processes that our cells are capable of.

Cardio exercise increases your chance of heart attack and premature death if done after age 40. A recent Mayo Clinic study following 3,200 people, starting when they were young adults, over a 25 year period, found that some people who exercised three times the national physical activity guideline were more likely to develop coronary artery calcification by the time they reached middle age; calcium-containing plaque that are present in the arteries in the heart are a predictor of heart disease.

There is no argument of the fitness benefits of incorporating physical activity in one's life. Our hunter-gatherer ancestors were most certainly physically active in order to survive (food acquisition, shelter maintenance). But this activity was not very strenuous; it was closer to walking then to jogging or running. Marshall Sahlins, a noted anthropologist, estimated that pre-agricultural hunter-gatherers spent about fifteen to twenty hours a week searching for food, in order to survive. Compare that to the Western work week of 40+ hours at work, then add in another dozen or two hours of commuting, and shopping for food and clothing, and household maintenance. Think about how much leisure time our ancestors had compared to our "affluent" society! This "exercise" only gave us better fitness, which is what mattered in evolution. It allowed us to survive; it did not increase longevity.

Probiotics

Just as Linus Pauling fraudulently promoted vitamins, we now have people fraudulently promoting probiotics.

There is such a thing as a person not having the correct type of bacteria in their digestive system. It is a hypothesis that the overuse of antibiotics has led to the increasing in the number of intestinal problems that modern humans now find themselves immersed with, problems such as ulcerative colitis.

There is a logical treatment for this. The "poop", or feces implant. A patient finds a poop donor and uses a douche to inject it into the rectum. This usually works short term, but rarely long term. It is not known why it does not work long term on everyone.

The medical industrial complex has attempted to make this a complicated process, telling us that only a few physicians in the world are licensed to perform this procedure. They want the donor to be screened for rare parasites and the poop to only be inserted into the anus by a specialist. Many patients have found donors on their own, bought generic douches, and performed the procedure successfully on their own.

Big pharma has teamed with physicians to make patients think this is a complex and dangerous procedure. So big pharma, and chemical and food manufacturers, created the probiotics market. Outside of helping to improve an occasional case of diarrhea, these products have been proven NOT to work as well as the bacterial flora occurring naturally in our gut, as they do not use the bacteria that naturally exists in our gut, and they have been linked to some nasty side effects such as bloating, gas, diarrhea, headaches, and SIBO (small intestine bacterial overgrowth).

There's an old saying; "there's a sucker born every minute". Once attributed to both WC Fields and P.T. Barnum, but now the author is officially unknown. This phrase applies to all who give in and purchase vitamins or probiotics in the belief that they "must" consume these products in order to be in line with their peers.

Gut problems often occur in waves in an individual, as do most illnesses. When the disease is on the down side, we attribute the diminishment of symptoms to what ever we were doing at the time. So if a patient takes probiotics and feels less symptoms, they give credit to the probiotics, which cannot aide you as they are not bacteria which normally live in a human!

I am sure many of you will spend a lot of money on probiotics instead of free poop.

Antibiotics Gone Wild

Do you use the liquid hand "sanitizers" in order to kill ALL germs?

Were you offered antibiotics every time you went to the doctors with an illness as a child?

Does your doctor still send you home with a prescription for antibiotics (154 million prescriptions are written annually, with 30% being completely unnecessary)?

Do US raised pigs, cows and chickens consume 130,000 tons of antibiotics annually?

The answer to all of these questions is "yes".

There has been a rapid emergence of resistant bacteria worldwide over the last decade, endangering the effectiveness of the existing portfolio of antibiotics in the physician's arsenal. As a result, bacterial infections are once again a threat. The medical industrial complex's overuse and misuse of antibiotics has led us into a potential crisis; it is now highly feasible that new strains of bacteria are out there that we will be unable to protect patients from.

The crisis actually started almost as soon as doctor's started prescribing antibiotics in the late 1940's, as the miracle drug that would save millions of lives during WWII was handed out by general practitioners like they were Tic Tacs. In the 1950's, penicillin resistant bacteria strains developed quickly, threatening most of the advances made in the 1940's. Big pharma reacted quickly by creating new antibiotics and quickly restoring the life-saving super powers of antibiotics. This too was short lived. This pattern has been repeated since then.

The major problem is a belief by the general public that antibiotics are a cure all and are necessary. We no longer let a little "illness" work itself out. We have been made to believe that we must go to the physician and that he must give us something in order for us to heal. The physician then feels pressured into giving their clients (patients) what they ask for as they want returning customers. And the overuse of the antibiotics is the result.

To add to this, most government funded facilities force an employee to get a "doctor's note" if they call out sick, in order to not be reprimanded or penalized. This forces an ill person (who would be fine staying home and resting while a 1-3 day virus worked its way out of them) to visit a doctor for a "note". The doctor will usually prescribe an antibiotic which is not needed and perhaps order additional and expensive unnecessary tests.

Today, over prescription of antibiotics has led to the development of superbugs; antibiotic resistant microbes.

And the use of antibiotics in livestock has been going on since the 1950's, to cause faster growth and decrease sickness. But they are most likely turning our livestock into superbug incubators. In 2013, a study determined that people living near pig farms or crop fields fertilized with pig manure are 30% more likely to become infected with staph infections.

Diabetes

Modern medicine educates patients who have blood sugar problems that Type 2 diabetes is preventable by a carefully regimented diet, and that Type 1 diabetes is incurable; that, once contracted, you are a life-long patient, dependent on insulin injections and periodic office visits.

Type 2 diabetes (adult onset diabetes) is a disease that you are told you can control if you come to the office regularly for blood and urine tests and maybe take a prescription only the physician can supply for you, and if you have regular consultations with their dietician. If not treated, it can cause blindness, foot amputation, and perhaps a shortened life span. The disease can be caused by either heredity or by lifestyle (lack of physical activity, a diet of high-fat foods and lacking in fiber, and obesity, which is often caused by the first two factors).

But there is an alternative.

For hundreds of years it has been known that starvation short of death, cures both Type 1 and Type 2 diabetes.

A 2011 study conducted by Newcastle University in England discovered (once again) that by practicing an extreme, low-calorie diet for two months, Type 2 diabetes can be reversed. The diet was limited to 600 calories per day and consisted of diet drinks and non-starchy vegetables, and was followed by a six month period of weight stabilization.

Another study demonstrated that starvation cured Type 1 diabetes.

Starvation has been shown to cure diabetes. When insulin was discovered and produced for sale, physicians turned to prescriptions instead of education, making themselves and big pharma even richer.

Name Brand Drugs are Superior to Generics

Anyone that tells you this is selling you a bad bill of goods. The name brand drug and its generic version both have the same API (active pharmaceutical ingredient; the chemical that delivers the drug's benefit) and both have similar bioavailability (the ability to deliver the API where it is needed). They are virtually identical, except for the name on their bottle.

Drugs are very expensive to develop. (The average cost was $2.6 billion for any given drug entering the market in 2018, an increase of $1 billion since 2003). As a result, drug companies are given a 20 year patent where they can market the drug without competition. This is why some drugs cost so much; as of 2018, there are over 20 drugs with a monthly cost of $25,000 or more available in the U.S. And who wouldn't find a way to come up with the $20,000 per year for meds to keep AIDS from killing you, or $84,000 to cure your Hep C?

But big pharma does some unethical practices when one of the drugs is approaching the end of their patent's life. Consider Nitrostat, a Pfsizer developed heart med. In late 2015, one year before the patent expired, the drug sold for $0.80/dose. A year later, after a series of price increases, the price had risen to $1.20/dose. Its generic, Nitroglycerin, entered the market at $0.95/dose, more than the brand name it was replacing was selling for just one year earlier! And one year after Nitroglycerin's launch, Nitrostat was selling for $1.75/dose.

Guess who sells Nitroglycerin? Greenstone LLC. Guess who own Greenstone LLC? Did you guess Pfizer? Correctomundo!

Another trick that big pharma does to maximize profits is to have the US subsidize the rest of the world. On average, for the top 20 meds accounting for 15% of global sales, the US pays 3 times more for the same med as the UK, 6 times more Brazil, and 16 times more for India, which is known as the country with the lowest cost meds in the world. Because the US medical industrial complex will pay big pharma what it asks for (remember, insurance companies stand to benefit from higher costs, since their profit is tied to revenue/premiums, provided they can predict their costs accurately and increase premiums accordingly), they can rely on basic supply and demand economics to determine how much other country's will pay for the same drugs.

And the worse news of all involves that big pharma has been colluding on generic pricing, costing the US billions. A federal lawsuit was filed May of 2019, involving 43 states against 13 pharmaceutical companies, covering 142 drugs, claiming conspiracy to fix prices.

Palliative (end of life) Care

We are all going to die

Death is a normal part of life, not a defect that a doctor must correct.

13% of America's spending on personal healthcare goes into palliative care, spent in the last year of a patient's life. And it's no wonder why this is so. As discussed previously in this book, we already have physicians that operate in an environment where they order a plethora of unnecessary tests and perform countless unnecessary procedures to be on the safe side. Nowhere is this practice more out of control then in a hospital where the patient is often in a life or death situation, exploiting our evolutionary drive to survive, squeezing out every additional minute of precious life from the patient, and buying the doctor their next Maserati. And if the patient has insurance (very likely, since we are usually dealing with Medicare-age Americans), the procedures are virtually free. And as any economist will tell you, when something is free, people tend to consume unlimited quantities of it.

What we fail to consider is the emotional cost of expending this financial expenditure. Consider the emotional cost to the family of keeping a loved one alive that has no brain functionality and zero hope of recovery, it's devastatingly stressful. Maybe there's hope here; 37% of Americans now have Advanced Directives, which dictates what is to be done to an incapacitated patient, including allowing them to die instead of having everything that could possibly be done to keep them alive from occurring. Thank science for AD's; they allow the patient to die, providing relief to their family and friends, and depriving the medical industrial complex from being able to squeeze every last cent out of a paying customer.

Earlier in this book, we discussed the treatment of cancers that will still result in the patient dying. Consider later stage lung cancer. Do you think that the patient hears the clinical facts as follows: "Option 1, aggressively fight your stage IV cancer? First, a four hour operation, with a four day hospital stay, with a six week recovery at home. Second, 24 weeks of chemotherapy. Third, seven weeks of radiation therapy. Likely outcome, 10 to 14% survival rate after five years. In summary, we'll spend a few hundred thousand dollars treating you, you'll feel like crap for the next nine months, start to feel better for three months, then quickly return to feeling like crap and dying three months later." Basically, choose this option and you'll live another 15 months, with 3 good months and 12 months of suffering.

Or, refuse treatment, in which case you die in eight months. You'll receive medicine to control the pain. It won't affect your lucidity for another 7 months, and you'll be out of it the last few weeks. So, ignore treatment and you'll only live another 8 months, but you'll have 7 good months.

And this doesn't even factor in the pain and suffering and inconvenience that you will put your family though with the treatment, them watching you near death for a year, than seeing hope for 3 months, only to see you go back to your death bed.

If we were explained our options in these terms, wouldn't it affect our decisions?

Unnecessary Removal of Body Parts

Knife happy doctors and dentists are cutting us up when it's not really necessary.

Appendixes A visit to the ER with a diagnosis of appendicitis almost guarantees the removal of the organ. And while there is little evidence that we still require the organ, a recent study (*Journal of the American Medical Association,* July, 2015) determined that 73% of all cases of appendicitis could be cured by antibiotics. Surgery would only be mandatory for cases involving more than inflammation (burst appendices, abscess, and tumors).

Wisdom teeth Human used to have 2-3 sets of wisdom teeth. It is not known why this changed over time, but this we know; our teeth have increased in size and our jaws have not. Now, as soon as a patient receives a diagnosis of one impacted wisdom tooth, even if it is not associated with any discomfort, the oral surgeon is brought in, removing not only the offending tooth but usually removing the opposing healthy tooth, and, in some cases, the two teeth on the other side of the mouth. Two UK 1998 studies (University of York and Royal College of Physicians of Edinburgh) both found that, unless patients have a condition necessitating removal (infection, tooth decay or cysts, damage being done to neighboring teeth, or severe pain), removal is unadvisable.

Breasts and ovaries As we begin to understand the human genome more, we introduce "solutions" to "potential" problems. With the discovery of the genes responsible for breast cancer, we now have women opting for a prophylactic mastectomy; the removal of their breasts as a preemptive strike against a disease that they are more likely to get then most women, but are not necessarily guaranteed to get. Women in the US are getting this procedure done to them. Research and proper data collection demonstrate that these prophylactic excisions serve no purpose. It was simply political correctness and a movie star promoting it to make the phrase "cut them off!" in vogue.

Penises Circumcisions occurred in as many as 40% of the global male population, as determined by the World Health Organization in 2011. Why did the parents of roughly over 1 billion baby boys opt to mutilate their sons against their will, inflicting pain on the newborn, when there is no good evidence for or against the procedure?

Orenstein's words about making women's body into time bombs can be related here. Doctor's and our society are making men look at their genitals as being "defective" if they don't have surgery on them.

Many men have committed suicide as a result of circumcisions gone wrong.

Alternative Medicine

Chiropractic Chiropractic is one of the largest expenditures in pseudo-sciences that Americans pump money into. At its foundation is the biggest unsolved mystery about chiropractic treatment, which is its practitioners being unable to explain exactly how spinal manipulation reduces back or neck pain, or any other ailment.

A recent study (*Spectacular Health*, Professor Edzard Ernst, February 18, 2016) discussed hundreds of cases in the UK of serious or permanent damage resulting from chiropractic adjustments. What's worse, only 23% of UK chiropractors report always discussing serious risks. Despite the industry being regulated (to which the author of the study comments that "even the best regulation of nonsense must result in nonsense"), the regulators noted a general disregard for the application of the precautionary principle of healthcare, which requires the practitioner to, whenever possible, utilize only those therapies which demonstrably generate more good than harm.

One study found a link between chiropractic manipulations of the neck and stokes cause by a tear in arteries in the neck, especially among people under 50. 9% of people suffering from this kind of stroke had a direct linkage to chiropractic manipulation.

Homeopathy Any process that is based on the doctrine of "like cures like" has no foundation in reality. It claims that any substance that causes the symptoms of a disease in a healthy person should cure the same symptoms in sick people. I'm not making this up!

From a scientific point of view, it makes tremendous sense why homeopathic medicines do not work. Homeopathic medicines are manufactured by highly diluting the "curative" substances which could have an effect in higher concentrations on the workings of the body. The substance is diluted so that it is practically impossible to find one single molecule of the "curative" ingredient. The "customer" is getting a placebo at best. Interestingly, the hucksters know this and claim that the curative substance doesn't need to be there; it has left its "influence" on the other substances in the "medicine". Anyone that has heard of chemistry knows that it is impossible for a chemical or element to leave an imprint. That's like saying that the air and water and plants and animals that we consume are themselves homeopathic medicines!

Acupuncture Acupuncture is based on Traditional Chinese Medicine, which, in tradition and practice, is self-admittedly not based upon scientific knowledge. The official Chinese word is that, even though they invented it, it doesn't work. They use it only as a tourism lure.

In a 2012 study conducted by England's National Health Service (who pays for acupuncture for one condition, the treatment of lower back pain) reported 325 patients that suffered complications, including dizziness (causing a total of 996 episodes of dizziness, with the patient losing consciousness in 63 of those instances), 5 cases of collapsed lungs, and 100 cases of needles being left in their bodies!

I am not against alternative treatments. Most of what "cures" us from a sudden problem works on the "placebo" effect. Most narcotics stop pain by this means. If a patient is left in a better state of mind after having had a water enema, or after having eaten a certain food, that is good. It is when we are told that we "must" accept a physician's treatment, "or you will die" that I disagree.

According the *Science Based Medicine (2013);*

1. Acupuncture is a pre-scientific superstition; it is based on Tradition Chinese Medicine and a concept known as qi involving a life force/vital energy that animates all living things.

2. Acupuncture lacks a plausible mechanism; any modern attempt to scientifically explain how acupuncture could work fails, including the possibility that the needles may stimulate the release of pain-killing chemicals, or that they relax tense muscles, or that block pain conduction.

3. Clinical trials show that acupuncture does not work; countless controlled clinical trials (using three groups; a control group receiving no intervention, a "sham" group experiencing needles placed in the "wrong" locations, and a "real" group) show no benefit from acupuncture.

Dental Matters

Do you brush?
Do you floss?
Gum disease, culture.

All work has the purpose of making money for the person performing the task. The cornerstone of capitalism is that everyone benefits only if we are all engaged in activities that are engaging with one another in mutually beneficial exchanges. But when customer/patients think they are receiving a song and dance, they lose faith in what is being done to them. And the medical industrial complex is no longer engaging in mutually beneficial exchanges; we, the customer/patient, are getting screwed over.

Remember our lawn company from earlier? They charge by the lawn. They do not measure each blade of grass and charge based on the height of the grass each time they service your lawn.

Dentists will measure your sulcus (depth of the ditch around your tooth and gums) and then come up with a confusing name and price they tell you must be carried out on you in order to prevent you from losing your teeth.

It is all the same. Whether 1 mm or 6 mm, the process is the same and does not justify a higher cost, but the hygienist will hide behind complexity, hit you will all foreign sounding terms and convince you that you must submit to the treatment or only bad things will happen to you. Problem is, dental organizations promote different dental codes for differing depths of pockets, introducing a new way for dentists to gain income, and help to justify the long hours and costs needed to achieve a dental degree. It all seemed great for the dental community. They "hide" behind complexity, or medical terms in order to convince you that you are not smart enough to decide these things on your own. But is it correct?

This falls into myths, fads and conspiracy. When dental insurance began, codes for a simple cleaning (prophy) were different than those for a debridement or scaling. So "voila!" a light is switched on in a dentist's head and there are no more prophys (simple cleanings that make your teeth feel smooth) administered to patients as they bring in the least amount of money, and usually they are "free" to the patient; they become scalings and root planings, which involve using sharp instruments supposedly to make your roots smooth, which bring in the most money. And scaling's have been found to cause attached gingiva (the firm gum that acts as a barrier to bacteria) to recede, or lower. But dentists ignore this fact and present the procedure to patients as something that "retains" this barrier.

Dentists will tell you gum disease causes heart problems because they heard that from a friend or salesperson and it sounds bio plausible. There is an "association" with gum disease and heart disease, but a cause has not yet been identified.

Recently a news story was released stating that there is evidence that an enzyme found in dental plaque is also found in the brains of Alzheimer's patients. For now it is just a story, but I am certain dental organizations have already handed out millions of pamphlets stating that gum disease causes Alzheimer's.

First, no research has been presented yet. Maybe an association will be found some day. If there is an association, a logical person might ask, if plaque causes Alzheimer's, and the rate of Alzheimer's has increased over the last century, how does that play into the fact that dentistry has pushed gum treatments for the last century?

It is much to the dental profession's advantage to not question this and just go with the flow. Much the same way that politicians over or under-stress "man-made climate change" if they think it gets them votes and power. The association or possible association of gum disease and

Alzheimer's works in the dentist's and dental association's favor as it gains them money and power.

I predict that in the future someone will make a connection with gum disease and Alzheimer's, and the politicians and the medical/dental world will go with it like a heated sled down a frozen mountain, and they'll be laughing all the way to the bank.

I would ask, if any disease is associated with gum disease, and the rates have increased as gum treatments have, wouldn't it seem likely that the gum "treatments" and not the gum "disease" is the cause?

Only time will tell if true research or politics prevails in this one as it has in many conditions before, all to our, the patient/customer's, detriment.

There is no dental prevention, only dental "preservation". Dentists can better preserve tooth structure if they treat early decay rather than waiting until a tooth causes pain or has visible decay (cavities). Makes sense. But that is NOT prevention.

Systemic fluoride does help prevent decay as the fluoride is then incorporated into the crystalline tooth structure while your tooth is soft and developing, from the time teeth appear to around six years of age. The topical applications you receive at the dental office provide very minimal prevention; the daily systemic dose you gave yourself at home as a child, when it would have been much more helpful to you, did make a difference. But fads and myths have led many to illogically fear fluoride.

Having your teeth cleaned in order to prevent decay and bone loss is bio plausible, but no evidence exists to support this. It is both cultural and a ritual. Patients expect to leave the office with smooth feeling teeth.

When a tooth is studied under the microscope, a pellicle, or thin slimy coating is found on the tooth. If you brush your teeth you can remove this coating, but never completely. Because of this, dentists, being scientists, justify brushing. But it is only bio plausible. There is no scientific evidence that it actually prevents decay or gum disease. Also, the smoothness of a root does not predict bone loss.

Same with flossing. No evidence that flossing prevents tooth loss, but it is bio plausible. And it gives the dentist and his staff something to stand for. Instead of you just coming into the office, having X-rays taken and the dentist looking at your teeth in order to preserve tooth structure, they can all talk to you, or rather lecture you on your brushing and flossing technique. It is in the dental culture, not scientific evidence.

It's all in the verbiage. It influences how you think and controls your priorities which deplete your emotional and financial capitol.

Fluoride

I don't know what the current myth with fluoride is today as it seems some groups always want to say something bad about it, such as;

- Fluoride in city water is a communist plot
- Fluoride causes cancer
- Fluoride is just bad for you
- Toothpaste without fluoride is better.

A recent observation in a Mexican town with a water supply containing an unusually high amount of fluoride had caused "fluorosis", a condition which causes teeth to turn brown. Government groups in the US decided that they should stop using systemic fluoride because one town in Mexico had high fluoride in its water.

Systemic fluoride has been the standard in fighting tooth decay for a hundred years. Its use is still recommended as the primary preventer of tooth decay. It is a naturally occurring mineral in our water supplies and is found all over the earth.

Unfortunately, the PC police and liberal government have convinced some medical and dental societies to not promote systemic fluoride anymore. Instead of the few sacrificing for the many, we now seem to be entering a society where the many are being told to sacrifice for the few. Because a few have had unnaturally high doses of fluoride and wound up with brown teeth, we must now all be subjected to subpar dental advice for the many to focus on treatment for the few.

I would prefer that my child had brown teeth that do not require dental drilling and extractions. Our current government say it is better to have white teeth even if it means losing them to tooth decay someday.

I will tell you this as a dentist and a scientist; I have seen it with my own eyes and it is well documented by correct research that the number one determinant of whether or not you get tooth decay, is whether or not you have fluoride in the crystalline makeup of your teeth. The only way to achieve this is by consuming fluoride while the teeth in question are soft and forming in your jaws.

If a pregnant woman ingests fluoride during her pregnancy, her child will not encounter tooth decay in its baby teeth.

If a child ingests fluoride between the ages of birth and 6 years old, he will not encounter tooth decay in his adult teeth.

There really is no way to prevent tooth decay other than the above. If you use oral fluoride and have not received systemic fluoride during tooth development, you will lessen your tooth decay, but will not prevent it. If you eat less sugar you will lessen decay, but not prevent it.

If you have sealants placed on your teeth and you did not ingest fluoride during tooth development, you will still get decay.

Public health organizations would not agree with me as they are political and want the population to think that they are acting in our best interests to get you to vote for their political party. First, they cause a "problem" (tooth decay) by stopping public water fluoridation projects (and the ignorant audience believes big government protected them from yet another harmful chemical), then they provide the "solution" (government subsidized topical fluoride and pit and fissure sealants, and restorations).

And while it's true that you will have less decay if you follow public policy, my gripe is that they have stopped advocating systemic fluoride which would solve the decay problem for 99% of everyone.

Periodontal (gum) disease

We have all been scolded by our hygienist and dentist to floss more, and floss better. We have been told if we do not floss we will lose all of our teeth to periodontal or gum disease. This myth has been promoted by dental supply companies who push a "soft tissue" program to dentists in order to sell their products which usually consist of magic tooth brushes.

But the cause remains the same; systemic inflammation. Dentists will tell you it is from "local" inflammation (meaning it originates due to debris in between the gums and the teeth). So dentists feel justified in scaling your gums every year.

Dentists also feel justified in treating gum disease due to their incorrect interpretation of the association of gum disease and heart disease. It is true the two are associated with one another, but the route of damage is reversed. Systemic inflammation leads to heart disease and gum disease. Dentists would like you to believe that gum disease causes heart disease since it is better for their bank account.

More recently, some "papers" have tried to blame Alzheimer's disease on gum disease. Of course, I do not know what real research will show about this, but I would bet dentists will pay back their dental associations by doing all they can to tie Alzheimer's to gum disease.

Dentists and physicians have chosen to ignore the observations which demonstrate that heart medicines and antibiotics that lower systemic inflammation have been observed to halt gum disease.

These dentists are blinded by the financial rewards of treating gum disease. As a result, they bait you by putting the fear in you that you will die sooner if you don't stop gum disease.

Gum disease is to dentistry as cancer is to medicine; a great big money generating machine.

Silver Fillings

Every decade or so, a discussion about silver fillings shows up in the news along with a new demon it unleashes on your body.

Silver or "amalgam" fillings were invented in the 1860's at the request of the US Army, to find a restorative material for teeth (fillings). The material had to be able to be stored without refrigeration and be easy to use in the field. The army has accurate and extensive records of all its personnel, including dental treatment.

The military physicians compared medical conditions of the millions of soldiers over 200 years who received silver filings with those who did not and compared the data. They found that there was no difference in a person's medical condition if they did or did not receive silver fillings.

But anti-military politicians welcome any suspicion that can cause our citizens to mistrust our military. It is all false, and I expect to see this misinformation in the news again soon. Amalgam or silver fillings have never caused an illness or medical condition in a person. (Anyone can have an allergic reaction to any substance).

Your dentist has no doubt tried to convince you to replace all of your silver fillings with a new-fangled amalgam, claiming the expansion and contraction of silver to hot and cold leading to tooth stress and cracking, or the leakage of mercury into your body, or just good old aesthetics. It's just the medical industrial complex looking for another way to sell you goods and services that you don't need.

Dental X-rays

Did you ever wonder why dentists place a lead apron on you when they take X-rays? I did. I was taught at my great dental school that it was only due to political correctness, and that in following this practice, your dentist was making you less knowledgeable and more paranoid about things that are not. Your dentist is allowing you to believe that dental X-rays are giving you cancer. As I stated earlier, radiation of any type has never produced cancer in anyone. Even government institutions have stated this. In Florida, for example, there is no requirement for the use of a lead apron while receiving x-radiation; not for pregnant women, not for anyone.

Very few dentists look into this, and I'm sure that 99% of dentists in Florida are not aware of this, or that radiation does not cause cancer.

Every 10 years or so, a major scare is created by the media. I don't know why, but it happens. Examples of these scares include salmonella in eggs, coca cola causing everything from cancer to diabetes, a linkage between vaccines and autism, mobile phones causing brain tumors, and blaming the increased consumption of high fructose corn syrup as the leading culprit in increased rates of obesity. These were all proven to be the media playing Chicken Little, running around saying that the sky was falling down. Be assured, there is no cause and effect of dental or any X-rays with cancer.

BUT! If a dentist were to not use a lead apron on a patient, they might lose that patient and get bad reviews on Yelp or Face Book or even have a law suit filed against them. They most likely would not lose, but the trouble, money and loss of reputation by an ignorant audience is too much for them to allow to happen. And if a patient developed some type of cancer, ANY type of cancer, there are attorney's that would take the patient's case, looking for anyone and everyone to sue that they could try to hold accountable for their client's cancer through their "malpractice".

A government website, in the past, was titled, "Why dentists use a lead apron when taking X-rays." It simply stated, "To save time on having to explain to the patient why it is *not* needed." So time trumps intelligence. I guess that that is the world that we live in these days.

Mental Health

One in six Americans take psychiatric drugs. That's over 50 million people! Sounds familiar? Remember, approximately 50% of our population is on blood pressure medicine.

We all behave differently, we all have different personalities. Physicians and socialists have managed to label different personalities as being the result of an illness. Now that these are illnesses, government healthcare insurers and others can lure you into buying their insurance and voting for their politicians so that they can "help" you.

Instead of a parent helping their child learn to concentrate more in school, big government has taken that responsibility away from the parents and put it on the state. Now there are "special" classes for these "difficult" personalities. There are psychologists who will diagnose your child, physicians who will medicate them. Adderall, Dexedrine, Metadate, Ritalin; any kid that can't sit still is put on one or more of these meds to "calm them down." Problem solved! Parents are off the hook.

And what of the current p.c. topic? Sex. If a person were to enter a psychologist's office and say that they thought they were Abraham Lincoln, the psychologist would most likely say the patient was having delusions and send them to a psychiatrist for further evaluation and therapy to bring them back into reality.

But. If your child told a school counselor they thought they were a girl when in fact they were a male, in some states, the counselor can help your child decided to surgically change their sex. And guess what? You, the parent, cannot stop this process or your child can sue you in court!

Our most liberal politicians, in an attempt to cater to citizens of all ways of thinking, have decided that in order to gain more votes, they will support those who have mental illness. This has led to a dangerous trend in many school districts, which are now shutting the parent out of deciding what to do with their children when the child notifies a school staff that they are having "delusions" of their sexuality.

Healthcare Center employees, which receive federal money, cannot tell a parent why their 12 year old had an appointment there. They can have a sexually transmitted illness, or receive injections of medicaments in their body, without the parent's permission! This is really happening NOW! IN the USA!

These children are being told not to change their outlook on life, but to change their physical bodies, with surgery and dangerous hormones. And while gender dysphoria is a scientifically proven condition, the majority of sex reassignment surgery patients had at least one psychiatric comorbidity in conjunction with their gender dysphoria (major depressive disorder, a specific phobia, and numerous instances of adjustment disorder, were the most common conditions) that remained after the surgery.

It seems very simple to half of our population that a delusion is a delusion. Not so to politicians. They want to put a specific diagnosis on all ways of thinking or acting in order to offer the public a cure that only the politicians can supply for them.

Many of our nation's heroes, if born today, would not have been heroes. They would have been categorized as having attention deficit disorder, or classified as narcissistic. They would not pass a military physical or psychological evaluation.

Instead of allowing differences in personality to blossom into something great, we medicate, then treat them into normalcy, into boredom.

Some well-known athletes have had their "super powers" dulled by mental health treatments. They had learned to use their different personalities to their advantage, until someone decided to convince them that they should seek psychological treatment and medicines which removed these advantages of personality and placed them in a category where they were considered to be "normal".

What if you have an addictive personality? Alcohol, smoking, and drugs are not the only things people get addicted to; doing anything so that it becomes an obsession is considered addictive, including eating, gambling, internet use, sex, exercise, shopping and work. Mental health professionals are quick to offer meds to limit the occurrence of some disorders, or reduce the discomfort associated with the behavior, or limit the symptoms to speed along recovery, and provide an easy solution for the many patients who are just looking for a quick fix, not treatment involving behavioral change (which is more likely to lead to a permanent fix). We have created the perfect feedback loop to expand the overuse of meds. It's no wonder there is an opioid addiction problem in the U.S. But what's worse, we might be overmedicating the next Thomas Edison or Henry Ford, diagnosing their high energy and creativity as ADHD!

If we nationalize healthcare (Medicare for all), which is the current path the U.S. is on, I am sure that all crime will be treated as a disease, and visits to spas, and hunger will be covered by socialized healthcare. The purpose is to justify the government in taking and controlling more of your money.

The opioid epidemic has become a major topic of news reporting as of late. But the over prescription of opioids goes back to the early 1990's, starting innocently from what was supposed to be temporary prescriptions for pain management following surgery. The combination of the addictive nature of these drugs (sometimes intensified by big pharma), and the source of the pain coming from subjective complaints (i.e., soft tissue damage) versus objective findings (i.e., broken bones), made it easy for a doctor to continue prescribing opioids to a patient. By the late 1990's, an estimated 100 million Americans had some kind of chronic pain. That was one-third of the adult population; that number must be subject to over estimation! The combination of people finding out about the ease with which one could get something to help them with any nagging ache that they had (just inflate the intensity of the pain to your doctor) as well as the good doctors wanting to ease their patient's pain, and the bad doctors looking for more customers, exacerbated the situation. Drug companies, working in cahoots with big government, jumped all over this increase in chronic pain, making opioids even easier to get. (Between 1991 and 2011, prescriptions for painkillers tripled, from 76 million to 219 million, reaching 290 million by 2016). And this epidemic is a uniquely American problem; our healthcare system has driven up premiums so high that many people choose plans with poor coverage. These plans encourage doctors to prescribe pills for chronic pain versus seeking a permanent cure (if the source of the pain is a broke/fix it situation). And in cases where the patients were found to be abusing their prescriptions, they were denied them, sending them to the black market, either purchasing the same drugs illegally or worse, seeking less expensive, more addictive illegal substances, like heroin. Heroin usage increased starting in the early 2000's, with heroin overdose deaths increasing by 286% from 2002 to 2013. And approximately 80% of heroin users admit to abusing prescription opioids before becoming heroin addicts.

Alas, even therapists have migrated away from being scientists in treating mental health and offering counseling, to being pseudo-scientists. During their education, therapists review the findings of randomized clinical trials covering the various disorders and conditions that they will be exposed to in their practices. These studies will show which treatments worked best with which patients. For years, therapists based their practices primarily on looking at the best treatment for a general condition as carried out in the studies, with some possible adjustments for patients that didn't fit perfectly into the studies. Some therapists occasionally preferred relying on either their personal experience, and/or discussing their patient's case with colleagues, seeking their colleague's experience, and designing treatment around this smaller and somewhat limited sample size. Over time, this form of treatment became more and more popular, and now it is more commonly used than looking at clinical trials; in 2013, the personal experience based treatment method overtook the randomized clinical trials method in the US. Today, you are more likely to get advice from your mental health professional based on a therapy that they have been using on a handful of patients that they "believe" is more effective, than a treatment proven to be the most effective after being used on hundreds of people with a similar condition.

Cognitive Behavioral Therapy (CBT) continues to be taught as the single best way in treating common disorders (namely, depression, anxiety). A 2009 meta-analysis conducted by leading mental-health researchers revealed that only 69% of American and British psychiatric patients received CBT. In a review of treatments for eating disorders, it was discovered that 30 percent were treated with "motivational work", and 25 percent with "mindfulness".

Pseudo-science has officially replaced real research in the field of mental health.

Stress

Stress. A vague term. What is it? Is it mental stress that you are aware of? Mental stress that you are not aware of? Is it of a physical nature, as when a person does not sleep for a few days on end? Is it a chemical stress as when a person is poisoned? What is it?

A psychologist would say it is a "perceived" stress, in other words, it depends on what a patients tells someone.

A biochemist might say it is a measure of cortisol in your circulatory system.

A trainer might say it is how much weight is placed on your muscles.

A lot has been written about stress lately, yet a lot is still not known about the role of stress in our lives. I do not know the answer, but I would like to digress for a moment and discuss stress from a quality of life point of view.

"Balancing stress" is one of those meaningless phrases such as "in moderation" or "balanced diet". Too much stress is said to lead to situations that sub-optimize your physical and mental well-being. And too little makes you lazy.

Just as there are many systems in the human body, there are many types of stress, and until these are clearly defined and measurable, it does little good to discuss them in an informative manner.

Consider our prehistoric ancestors. Humans, like most animals, have a natural response to a stressful situation; it's called fight or flight. Imagine, it is 50,000 years ago, and you are wondering down a path to gather some food. A saber tooth tiger comes out of nowhere and plants itself in front of you. Your body's response; your cortisol and adrenaline flows, your heartrate and blood pressure soar, your muscles tense, even your narrow focus expands from food gathering to survival. In the next few minutes, you will either live (throw rocks at the tiger, climb a tree, run like the wind) or die. If you live, you will return to your normal mental and physical state in no time. You will learn from the experience and attempt to avoid it in the future. Your body and mind will benefit from the event. And hopefully, you will reproduce someday, and have little cave babies that have your great ability to thrive and survive under stress.

If you die, you will not reproduce, and natural selection will do its job.

Generalist-Specialist Ratio

In the United States, 20 to 30% of doctors are generalists and 70 to 80% are specialists. It is the exact opposite in the rest of the developed world. RBRVS (Resource-based Relative Value Scale) is used to determine how much money medical providers should be paid. The system was developed by Harvard University in 1985 and was adopted by Medicare in 1988. Today, it is still used by Medicare in the United States and by nearly all health maintenance organizations (HMOs). This has had three impacts on healthcare costs and practices:

1. Physician revenue (patient expenditure) is based on effort rather than effect. This encourages the overuse of both complicated procedures and endless tests, without consideration for outcomes.

2. Since the medical value of their service to the patient is disconnected to how much is paid, there is no incentive to either reduce the patient's cost or to actually help the patient.

3. And since the revenue potential for a physician shifts toward having a specialty (specialists generally take home twice the pay of generalists), an imbalance of generalists to specialists results.

Because the AMA (American Medical Association) offers significant input into the systems ongoing revision, and because the AMA is dominated by specialists, it has done the public a huge disservice of both limiting the overall number of seats in medical schools (we rank 9th of 11th industrial countries in doctors per 100,000 people) and by encouraging doctors to becoming specialists. The CMS (the Centers for Medicare and Medicaid Services), which administers Medicare, is also a major culprit in the misuse of this data. And since the United States is on a course toward socialized medicine, and there is a high probability that it will be Medicare for All, it is crucial that we change this process ASAP.

Living Forever (or at least to 100)

The life span of humans has not increased significantly in the 200,000 plus years that Homo sapiens have roamed Earth. Median life expectancy has increased; reductions in traumatic deaths and infant mortality, and the discovery of anti-biotics and vaccines are the major contributors. But most of the improvements have happened since 1950. The Great Depression and World War II temporarily set back many of the gains made in the industrial area, but the continued industrialization of the planet should get rid of the differences in life expectancy between the developing world and modern societies.

Unfortunately, median human life spans have only increased marginally in 200,000 of existence. Unless we can do something to change the aging process, peak human life span will stay at around 95 years old. And you will generally have to have won the genetic lottery to be able to make it to 95 and not have inherited any of the genetic tendencies (toward cancer, chronic lower respiratory disease, accidents, stroke or cerebrovascular disease, Alzheimer's disease, diabetes, influenza and pneumonia, kidney disease, and intentional self-harm or suicide) to even get that far. But there remain a slew of major factors impacting aging, including a number of routines involved at the cellular that have to be tackled before we are able to get life spans into the 100's.

And we have barely scratched the surface of these cellular level processes. Some progress toward reversing these processes has been made in mice (by tweaking genes that turn adult cells back into embryonic-like cells) show promise, but we are a long ways off.

And what would be the purpose? If we don't change the healthcare system soon, we'll just wind up with more years as a paying customer, making the medical industrial complex richer while we deplete our financial and emotional capital.

ATTITUDES

The medical industrial complex has put us in the current situation that we find ourselves, one where healthcare has gone wild, due to two primary issues; we abandoned both test pilots and science, and we went from being patients to being customers in the process.

Our institutions

We have many clubs that are referred to as "associations" or "societies". These in fact are simply clubs who have, as their primary goals, the continued existence of that corporation, along with the maximization of their shareholder's wealth.

Corporations are run by a Board of Directors that "directs" the CEO and their executive team, whose primary task is generally the maximization of shareholder wealth (make more money and increase the value of the corporation; increase the share price). In order to do this, they seek opportunities to increase revenues, usually by developing new products and services, while decreasing costs. In the case of corporations within the medical industrial complex, they are constantly developing new goods (pills) and services (procedures) by "inventing" bio plausible health "problems" that the customer needs to address in order to increase the human experience. Physicians, dentists and patients/customers ravenously consume these innovations. Following these practices and policies is to our detriment.

Instead of your physician giving you an answer to your latest health related question with "valid research demonstrates this treatment helps", they simply say "the _____ Dental Association" or the "_____ Cancer Society" recommends it.

And politicians eat this up as they receive donations from these organizations and then, in turn give the organization political power by insisting that government money goes to causes recommended by them.

One hand washes the other.

These associations/societies, do not have the ultimate correct answer or best research at their disposal, nor are they the authority on medical/ dental procedures. Their priority is maximizing political power, not ensuring your medical well-being.

We no longer know what research is

This phenomena started decades ago. Students with doctorate degrees in science could not discern between a real research paper and an essay written by someone with an agenda.

For instance, studies that were well carried out and critiqued by science editors, then published in very discerning science journals, are now referred to in more current research of the same subject. So, they are not only committing poor science, they are committing plagiarism! And no one seems to care!

Worst of all, this type of ignorance continues on at break neck speed.

Subjects such as longevity and blood pressure, once the focus of actual research, are now written without the authors performing a literature review. And this is indicative of our youth putting whatever they want on the internet and then patting themselves on the back, telling themselves they discovered the most important thing in history (*Healthy Says Who?*).

Not only do they think they are geniuses, but they also ignore important data and conclusions that would completely discredit their "research".

Essays sold as "research" are now no more than simple amateur essays published in order to get "likes" rather than to demonstrate actual research.

We no longer have test pilots

As stated earlier, the test pilot plays a crucial role in the design and use of a military airplane. Medicine and dentistry used to be filled with test pilots. But today, the medical industrial complex has all but abandoned this practice.

Consider the history of the smallpox vaccine, the first vaccine ever developed. It starts in 1796, when physician/scientist Edward Jenner observed that milkmaids who had previously been infected with the cowpox did not later catch smallpox. He devised an experiment that demonstrated that exposing subjects to cowpox protected them from getting smallpox. Although the first vaccine was nothing more than cow puss teaming with virus, it was effective.

Before the vaccine came into being, smallpox had a mortality rate of 35%, killing hundreds of thousands in the 18th century. The vaccine quickly became required in Western Europe. Unfortunately, it left much room for improvement, as there was a small chance of contracting syphilis using the "arm to arm" method, and the virus actually mutated during the 19th century. But science perfected the vaccine (especially after the germ theory of disease was solidified in the late 1800's). A global effort eradicated the disease by 1979 (1949 in the US).

We will need scientist-test pilots to face the upcoming challenges in the 21st century, be they tackling the next epidemic brought on by our overuse of antibiotics, treating illnesses at the cellular level, changing our approach to find ways for people to live with cancer (versus playing Mr. Potato Head with them), treating dementia with stem cell therapy, as well as the opportunities to develop medical scanners (a la *Star Trek*) to quickly diagnose patients, gene editing to eradicate genetic diseases, or lab grown replacement bones.

The birth of political correctness and the end of the accurate transfer of information

It is difficult to determine when and why our country became so obsessed with political correctness. Maybe it was born out of the political right, during the McCarthy years, when lives were ruined seeking out the communists among us. Maybe it was born from the political left, from the counter-culture movements of the 60's captured in *Steal this Book*, or the Occupy Wall Street movement. Maybe it was born out of both, with the publication of *Rules for Radicals*, a template used by the likes of both Jesse Jackson and the Tea Party. Regardless of its official origin, it has gotten to be such an issue that even universities, which were always the one place where the free flow of ideas was encouraged, are now having to worry about what is taught and who is allowed to speak at events. This culture of political correctness is hampering the free flow of ideas.

I take part in many forums about my medical problems. I ask questions and criticize.

While recently participating in two such forums, I was banned as I apparently hurt someone's feelings. So you see, if physicians will not consider a question or alternative idea, or a criticism, then how will we further medical treatment? This is the reason why properly conducted research is subjected to a peer review process.

In one forum, I posed the following question; "Does anyone have any properly conducted research that demonstrates that lowering blood pressure actually increases life span?" I received one response of, "I will not even address that question", then was banned from the site the next day.

On a Crohn's disease forum, I was banned for suggesting that physicians were more concerned with performing colonoscopies than in helping their patients within a week of ruffling their feathers.

I am proud of being banned from these fragile physicians' forums. These are the so called professionals who are treating us. They will only push their agenda and cannot tolerate someone who questions them. And this is hurting your treatment!

But all the fault is not with the physicians; patients are also to blame.

Many of these ignorant physicians are pressured into giving ignorant patients what they want. Patients often don't know what they need as they are manipulated by high pressure sales techniques into accepting treatments, so they become angered if the physician does not give them what they desire. Their desire is fueled by what they see in the media. Patients have become consumers, and bad consumers at that, seeking the easy way out and being manipulated by the goods and services that the medical industrial complex is pimping.

Consider the way that we decide if a physician is a "good" physician. We ask our friends, who know nothing of science or medicine, or we refer to public opinion in reviews. It all means nothing except that we value opinion over facts.

Patients are selfish and want what they can acquire for free from their insurance companies. Physicians and dentists want patients to continue to visit them. The patients think they are beating the system by getting things for free. The doctors want to make money so they do not discourage the patients from doing this, even if they know it is unnecessary.

Popularity is just popularity. Some physicians who have performed the most procedures have been found guilty of malpractice numerous times in courts of law. Some are popular because they advertise that they will get the "most" out of your insurance for you (they will punish the big bad insurance companies in order that you get the most procedures paid for you by them). Maybe their parking lot is always full because of the many misinformed patients frequenting their practice. To the patient "shopping" for a new doctor, this means that the physician must be good. This approach might hold true for a restaurant, but is not the right way to evaluate a medical practice!

Politicians do the same. They find or create a situation that you want solved (such as creating a fear that a certain food causes cancer), then tell you that only "they" can solve this problem for you by lobbying for more money, or regulating you.

This creates a situation where we are all swayed or are pushed into putting importance on popularity and consensus rather than on the truth.

Headaches

So you have a headache. Throbbing, stabbing pain that is almost unbearable. I put this topic here because if a dentist ever needs the skills of Wallace, it is in the case of headaches.

Physicians used to have a description of headaches called "migraine" headaches. They assumed there was a mysterious entity which caused intense headaches that caused pain behind the eyes, sometimes in the neck and back, and at other times caused blurred vision and dizziness which could lead to nausea.

Dentists argued that there was no such "entity" and finally, in the 1980's, the use of the term "migraine" was put to rest. There is no "mysterious" force or entity which causes intense headaches. There are only intense headaches and their complications which arise from the forces of the jaws. Adding ignorance to patient's understanding of medicine, some physicians continue to use the term "migraine".

It takes a dentist of great knowledge, experience, and bedside manners to care for such a problem. Few of these exist in our current dental system today.

The most common cause of a headache is from the jaw muscles clenching. The dentist must be sure that this is the cause, not a bad tooth, or brain tumor, or broken jaw. This is accomplished by observation, questioning, and X-rays if they feel they will be of value.

Dr. Wallace would take about five minutes to evaluate and treat this.

What is causing the clenching? Is it from thoughts? Or teeth that don't bite correctly? What is the solution that is the fastest, cheapest, and causes the least amount of side effects?

What do current dentists do? They first think about what their colleagues would do, then about a future law suit, then what will make them the most money.

So a simple night guard and muscle relaxant instead becomes a visit to a neurologist, oral surgeon and perhaps to a psychologist, all while the patient is suffering in extreme pain and missing work. Not to mention that they are suffering from additional stress by the physician making them believe that they might have cancer.

So what have we become?

Your Right to Live in the Reality of Your Choice has been Shanghaied!

Watch any TV station and you will be inundated with commercial after commercial of pharmaceutical companies threatening your health if you make one wrong decision on a medication you might be taking, or other propaganda by law firms telling you that, "An operation or medication you were prescribed could be life threatening, so call us and you might receive millions of dollars".

All of the above prevents you from having freedom of thought. The propaganda demands that you think about everything you do with your body. You must eat this, go to a specific doctor, have a test your doctor did not prescribe, remember what material was used in your surgery, and even though you feel great, "maybe" you will experience great medical problems soon, or even "death"!

We have all been shanghaied by fear and insecurity by the medical and dental professions.

Our founding fathers are said to have been both "free thinkers" and libertarians. They lived by the thoughts that we are all born, live, and die, and that we all have the right to do as we wish with our lives, that we each had the right to spend our emotional and financial capital as we chose to, providing we do not infringe on others in the process.

Today, we are told that we must micromanage every aspect of our life. That we cannot sit outside and breathe fresh air, look at the sky and feel good, or enjoy life on this planet. All media demands that you use your emotional capitol on stressful ideas. The media exploits the natural human practice of looking for bad things, dangers in our environment that could cause us harm, and pushes "bad news" at us 24/7. If it bleeds, it leads.

Our founding fathers were libertarians. They believed in protecting your right to live in the reality of your choice. Now there is very little we can do that is freedom of choice. Big government has crept into all aspects of our lives and we should all be upset with this.

If a depressed, ill person wants to take their life, they are a criminal. If you find a food or herb that you can consume that puts you in a state of mind you find pleasing, you are a criminal.

The USA is the freest country in the world, yet its citizens have allowed corrupt, nanny state leaning liberals, and progressive denying conservative politicians to take almost all of our freedoms from us.

Record Keeping

Part of the "why" of why physicians and dentists mismanage patients is record keeping. It is not an excuse, but from my experience, it is very difficult to overcome.

Physician's and dentist's job security is dependent on how their records are kept. This has been exaggerated with the intrusion of more government in making more regulations and wanting to have government hands in the medical/dental business. Record keeping is now all electronic, not to help the patient, but to aide government workers in being able to find a violation in record keeping.

In this new and "improved" method of electronic record keeping, you are simply a category. A button that must be clicked in order to prevent a physician from receiving a bad score from the government. Not only dentists and physicians, but nurses and other medical staff now use most of their time on the job (which should be used in treating patients) and experience in clicking buttons. Instead of being rewarded for good diagnosis and treatment of patients, they are rewarded for clicking buttons.

Instead of the emphasis being on what was done to the patient, the emphasis is on what you clicked on a computer program. It is a result of clinician's medical training and the desire for liberal, big government politicians to want to control what the physicians and dentists do. Medical and dental students got where they are by being competitive to get the best grades or scores. That competitiveness now equates to computer clicks. It is in their DNA, to compete.

Not all people will die from tuberculosis, or Ebola, but all patients are treated as if they will.

Data does show that some patients will die from the above, so being a hypochondriac is justified.

NO one has ever been found to have died from high blood pressure, or to have been saved from death by lowering their blood pressure. Two very good research projects demonstrated this. So WHY is everyone checked for high blood pressure, and why is 50% of the US population medicated in order to lower their blood pressure?

These computer record keeping programs are morphing into intrusions in the physician's and dentist's diagnosing and prescribing abilities as some will not permit a clinician from going to the next page unless they "click" that they have performed or prescribed what the "program" said they must. The politicians assign political allies to run the offices that control medical insurances and they believe that they are more educated, or have more of a "right" to dictate what a physician or dentist does. It is a very dangerous and autocratic path we are being led down, and we are ALL guilty of allowing this to occur.

Clinicians in the past wrote their observations, diagnoses and treatments on a piece of paper. Computer records were meant to simply replace a digitized piece of paper. Now they serve to remove power from the physician and dentist and to give it to a political ally.

We are no longer healers

"Hello sir, what ails you?"

I expect this to be your greeting at any medical office. Instead you hear, "It's time for your exam. Why did you miss your last one?"

Physicians are supposed to be here to "heal" you, to fix that which ails you or takes away from your quality of life.

Our politicians have now moved everyone's focus to the "business" of medicine rather than on "healing".

What was The Affordable Care Act? Was it a system to encourage better diagnosis and healing methods? No! It was a system which forced citizens to look at insurance companies as being evil, and government as being good. It had nothing to do with making people better able to enjoy their lives. And it had nothing to do with bringing down the cost of healthcare. It was all about making insurance premiums more affordable by a combination of government subsidies and mandating that everyone has to take out coverage. We basically passed the subsidies onto the taxpayer (in the first case) and the youth (in the second case, forcing them to pay for insurance). As a result, 30 million more customers that will consume unlimited quantities of "free" (to them) healthcare have been created for the medical industrial complex to exploit, increasing demand, while supply remains relatively fixed, thus driving costs up.

Our physicians now must focus their attention on things like hand sanitizer, antibiotic pre-medication, unnecessary tests and surgeries. Which works out great for them; they have more customers with money to spend.

If physicians did have a "motto" it would be that, "The earlier you test and find an ailment, the longer you will live". It is no longer, "First, do no harm."

If the above is true, then why not have all citizens have a full body MRI every 6 months? I do not know the answer to this. But it must benefit politicians in some way.

Or, is this the next miracle cure that the ACA's is going to force upon us in their quest to create preventive medicine?

Human success

I propose the following questions to you;

How do you define human success? How do you want to spend your life?

I define human success as "being able to live your life in the reality of your choice" (*Understanding Why*, Naryshkin).

So, what is the reality you envision for your life? Is it one where you want to spend all of your emotional and monetary energy (capitol) on searching your body for cancer? A search which will penalize you in some way (surgical scaring, loss of body parts, radiation poisoning, chemical poisoning)?

Or a life where you enjoy your time with friends, family and hobbies that you love and enrich your existence?

Our emotional capitol

I, like most people, set money aside for safe keeping. In order to do this, I have to live on a budget, allocating funds for housing, food, vacations, gifts, etc. I certainly do not want to use any for negative experiences such as being placed in a near death situation, or to use it on something I will never use or need, or to search for something that will result in negative feelings.

I also suggest that we all have an "emotional" capitol budget, a reservoir of thoughts and feelings. We only have so much to use. I hope to use mine on things that make me and my family happy. I would not want to use my emotional capital on negative things, such as being in a heightened fear of death, or worrying about my fitness.

But that is exactly what many of us choose to voluntarily use our financial and emotional capital for. Most of us are concerned with health insurance, and with keeping our annual or semiannual exams at our physicians and dentist's office. You think it is imperative that you have your teeth cleaned, or your blood pressure taken, or blood drawn, or have cameras stuck in all variety of orifices.

And when we have those things done to us, we suffer with the fear of the doctors finding something "bad", and that somehow makes us feel good?

Human beings have existed in some form for four million years. We did not think about what we ate, or if we had to get the advice of someone about our bodies. Humans lived long lives thousands of years ago, long before we became "civilized", as evidenced in archeological records, in a time when doctors, dentists and pharmacists did not exist.

These fears that the medical industrial complex uses to steal both your emotional and monetary capitol are fads which were created by misinformation by the medical industrial complex, big government, and the media.

Once again, we are reminded of the old saying, "There's a sucker born every minute".

Flying by the seat of our pants

In the early days of aviation, pilots flew by their instincts. Sophisticated instruments were not available or were not in wide use. Even in the late 20th century, military pilots were trained in "contact flying", which was using your instincts, rather than instrumentation, in order to have an instinctive feel for the plane. (This would be essential if they ever lost instrument readings in flight.) We looked out the windscreen at the horizon in order determine the aircrafts attitude, rather than looking at the artificial horizon (an instrument) in the cockpit. We looked at the earth to determine where we were rather than use navigation instruments. Modern military pilots continue to be trained this way.

In medicine and dentistry, we *were* trained similarly to military pilots. When a patient was presented to us in school, we were taught to observe their behavior and appearance. We were taught to carefully listen to their complaints. Using our knowledge, observing the patient's behavior, and conducting a physical examination, we would come up with a diagnosis of their condition. We then looked at laboratory tests, including X-rays to confirm our diagnosis, or tell us nothing, before prescribing a course of treatment.

Fast forward to current times and see that all of this has been thrown out the window.

When a patient presents to a practitioner in today's world, the patient is seen as a customer. The first question that the office staff asks is what insurance they have? Then a computer searches to see what tests can be run and what their insurance will pay for, and the tests are ordered. Surely they will not object to a test if it is not costing them anything?

Then the practitioner waits for test results in order to come up with a diagnosis. (Most of the time, the tests will tell the physician what is wrong with the thing it tested, but not always what ails the patient.)

Consider a patient with upper respiratory problems, which includes sore throats and colds. These could be categorized based on a patient's behavior and symptoms (what the patient tells the practitioner) and epidemiology (what is occurring in the population now?). Now the practitioner first thinks of how they can turn this encounter into money for the practice.

A simple virus, or an allergic reaction, which could be diagnosed properly over the phone. The customer will be required to come to the office (where the average time a typical customer has to wait from the time they contact the office to the appointment is 29 days!), followed by waiting an average of 41 minutes to see the doctor, who will spend an average of 11 seconds allowing the customer to explain what is wrong with them before interrupting, while only spending an average of 13 to 16 minutes with the customer! The customer is filled with fear as the doctor lists all the horrible diseases that they could have. Then the doctor lists all the tests that need to be run in order to determine what ailment the customer has. They take a nasal swab test to determine if it is a virus, then throat swab to determine if it is bacterial. These tests can run into thousands of dollars, but don't worry, your insurance will pay for them.

Then you have to wait anxiously for the test results which will "inform" the doctor what is wrong with you and what actions need to be taken to "heal" you.

Another example; a male child with abdominal pains walks into a pediatric office with his mother. Instead of the physician questioning the mother about the child's diet, the doctor elects to solve the problem by running expensive stool exams, followed by a colonoscopy. And the only thing that is probably wrong with the child was that he was constipated, most likely from a something he ate, and the only treatment he probably needed was a glass of prune juice. (This actually happened to my son recently). The doctor started listing off all of the things that my son might have wrong with him followed by a list of expensive, evasive and time consuming tests that they wanted to run, including an invasive, dangerous and expensive colonoscopy!) I refused all of the physician's advice as being completely idiotic and gave my son some prune juice, and voila! The simplest explanation for his discomfort turned out to be the correct one (constipation)! And no prescriptive medications were needed.

You, being a citizen of the planet, look at our modern information network every day, and are bombarded with incredibly horrible stories which might not even be true, filling you with massive anxiety. You don't want to be one of those horrific stories. You buy into the fear and agree to everything, thinking that if you have one of these ailments, you must use the shotgun blast approach and hit it with as many projectiles as you possibly can, and only then will you "win". You can determine your destiny if you have the right insurance that will allow for expensive and intensive tests and treatments.

By the time your lab tests arrive, your symptoms have gone away, but you will gladly take the expensive medications the doctor prescribes because maybe the deadly bugs are still hiding in your body.

Very few of us contract bacterial infections, but suggesting to a patient that they "might" contract an infection achieves the greatest monetary returns for the practice. And keeps them out of court defending frivolous law suits.

An allergy or simple virus is presented as a possible "strep throat infection".

Back pains will mysteriously remedy themselves in 6-9 months. If you choose to go to a physician and permit them to go on a treasure hunt, they will take X-rays and MRIs. These have been proven to not diagnose the causes of back pain (in the case of soft tissue damage; sprains, strains, muscle overuse) but if you buy into his fantasy of search and destroy, you will be put through major surgery, or have your back manipulated and perhaps damaged more by a chiropractor.

Again, it is due to a physician not being able to use their diagnostic ability (or lack of) and, instead, resorting to costly tests and then putting you through procedures which they can justify from the results of the lab tests.

Norman Hadler wrote, "We have great surgical techniques and surgeons. The problem is that these surgeries are being performed on patients who don't require them."

Much of unnecessary surgery that is performed is a result of a patient demanding it simply because they feel that if their insurance pays for it, they should receive it. So your physician is giving you what you want as long as they can fudge the diagnosis with the aid of costly lab tests. So you are happy, and they are happy.

But is it correct?

The physician's priority was their well-being in the form of their bank account, not yours. They won't take a chance to treat you correctly, via the "flying by the seat of your pants" method. They must treat you according to their social status, "what if" fears, and law suit avoidance.

I am sure you have purchased an item and the cashier could not give you change if they did not have a cash register program that calculated the change for them. In the same way, computer records and extensive testing where the lab creates a diagnosis for the physician have turned your doctor into an automaton, and now they cannot diagnose or use common sense in diagnosing and treating you. Physicians would benefit greatly if they spent three months out of every five years in clinics in developing countries where technology is not a given, forcing them to become real scientists again, and fly by the seat of their pants.

Superstition

Superstition is the act of repeating an act and expecting a result based on your performing this act before, even if the act did not actually cause the result you achieved.

This occurs more in dentistry than medicine, but it still occurs. If one were to visit 10 dental offices and study the chemicals, impression materials, drills, needles, anesthetic, etc. that each office used, you would see they ALL have different materials and supplies. If you were to ask each dentist WHY they use what they do, they would either be stone faced or they would tell you that their materials work best, or yield the best results.

In fact, the dentist just happened to get a desired result and attributed it to a specific material and now they swear by it, when, in fact, it had nothing to do with their success. Although, in dentistry, there are often thousands of ways and products that can solve the same problem, and most are correct. This behavior is found all over medicine and dentistry and patients often suffer as a result.

Physicians and dentists have become consensus seekers, rather than seekers of knowledge. They want to be accepted, and have allowed that need to override their purpose of finding the scientific truth.

Physicians are forced to use superstitious practice imposed on them by health insurance companies, big pharma, their malpractice insurers, and medical appliance companies. Consider the case of hip replacement surgery. Orthopedic surgeons are required to have a representative from the company that is providing the artificial joint in the operating room, driving the cost of the procedure up substantially. (Supposedly, this practice ensures that the right size joint will be used.) No other country in the world has this requirement. This is one of many reasons why this procedure costs an average of $40,000 in the U.S. and only $12,000 in the U.K.

In the practice of mental health, we previously discussed the fact that the majority of practitioners currently rely on their personal, limited experience and their colleague's experiences instead of relying on clinical studies of thousands of patients. One could argue that relying on personal experience is more akin to superstition when clinical data is available.

Justification by Statistics

I promised myself in writing this book that I would not use my experience as a patient as an example, but in this case, I think it makes this section clearer.

I was diagnosed with ulcerative colitis. I was diagnosed from symptoms and X-rays. My gastrointestinal specialist wanted to verify my condition with a colonoscopy and endoscopy. These were explained to me as being mandatory tests. When asked the justification for this, I was told that a patient that has ulcerative colitis has a 3% greater chance of having colon cancer.

Let's think about this logic. If a patient does not undergo a colonoscopy in his lifetime, he is an unknown. He dies an unknown to colon cancer. The statistician puts him on the chart as a person dying who did not have colon cancer.

From earlier, I explained that 50% of UC studies have shown NO higher risk of having colon cancer, so why aren't we making colonoscopies optional instead of forcing patients into an invasive procedure and worrying them about having cancer?

The majority of patients who have been told that they "might" get cancer will follow their physician's recommendation to the "t", fearing death from cancer. Full body MRIs are not recommended by many medical organizations as they show many illnesses or oddities that will never effect the patient's life, as well as often yielding false positive results that will imply the existence of a life-threatening illness, putting the patient into a frenzy, and generating a battery of additional tests to rule out the miss-diagnosis. But the practitioner must identify and tell the patient about the results or risk being sued down the road. Now the patient, who would have lived a normal, fit life, spends their life living in fear of dying from some horrible disease.

So a patient who is told to have annual colonoscopies will follow instructions. If a sign of cancer does show up, this patient's life is essentially ruined; they become a chronic cancer patient and undergo radiation therapy, chemotherapy, and perhaps surgical removal of their intestines, and spend the rest of their life emptying a colostomy bag.

Some life, eh? They will be listed by the statistician as a colon cancer patient.

If the same patient never listened to their doctor, they would have lived a normal happy life except for potentially having some occasional diarrhea. They die as a non-cancer patient.

BUTTTT. The physician will use the incorrect data that ulcerative colitis patients have a higher probability of developing cancer as an excuse to perform an expensive colonoscopy each year, gaining the approval of colleagues, while adding a second Mercedes in their garage!

What we are to the physicians

When medical students enter medical school, many students have a feeling that they are embarking on a noble cause. They envision helping the needy, saving lives, and freeing patients from pain.

Then they enter the medical industrial complex and learn that "quantity" of life is emphasized over "quality".

What are we to physicians now?

To most physicians and healthcare workers, we are simply CUSTOMERS!

We walk in the door and we are eyed by the staff. Are we trying to get a free exam? Are we trying to get narcotics to support an addiction? What is our insurance situation? Do we seem to be easy to convince?

The physician's focus is not on healing you. Rather, their focus is on how they can turn you into a life-long patient/customer, and on how they can best document what they think a potential future jury will want to hear in order to have the physician NOT be found guilty of committing malpractice on you.

They use this way of thinking when ordering very expensive X-rays and blood tests, and whatever else your insurance will pay for, because, how could you say no? How could you possibly object? They easily talk you into "taking advantage of your insurance".

If you question their reason for the tests, this only strengthens their decision on ordering them; they suspect that if you question anything they say, you might be the litigious type, all the more reason for ordering tests to cover their ass.

And this line of reasoning makes both their practice and the labs they refer their patients to, much richer. So it is a win-win situation all around as far as the medical industrial complex is concerned.

Instead of thinking about how they can heal you, they are thinking about what insurance you have and what codes they must use in order for their office to receive the most money. I call it "hiding behind complexity". You are hit with medical jargon and given a grim review of what you might have or might contract in the future.

"It's your fault! You didn't take your medicine! You didn't brush your teeth every day! You didn't watch your diet!"

I don't know if you have all been lectured to by a physician, a dentist, or their staff at some time. It is all part of the great manipulation that creates a feeling of guilt with the patient if they do not do as told and that they are somehow letting the practitioner down if you do not follow these orders.

Coding and computers

Coding is the way in which a medical doctor or their office charges you, or, most likely, your insurance company. If the service they provided to you is not listed in the official medical code, they cannot receive monetary funds from that company for that procedure.

Regardless of your political affiliation, we should all be supremely disappointed in the process that our government went through in bringing about the Affordable Care Act. More importantly, it was the process that they didn't use, namely, the use of the Congressional committee process. (This process ensures that a complicated issue will be explored in great length, and that experts will testify to ensure that Congress has all of the data they need in order to draft the bill. The ACA was done hastily, and was not bi-partisan, and we the citizen suffer and continue to suffer as a result. The republicans did the same thing with the tax reform of 2017.)

Medical coding is one of the least thought out provisions of the ACA that has led to serious issues involving medical billing. Overall, the ACA has made the medical billing processes significantly more complicated, which has forced many medical practices to outsource their medical billing, driving up healthcare costs, and, therefore, driving up healthcare premiums. But more seriously is how the ACA changed some coding for political reasons. The perfect example of this involves breast cancer.

As stated earlier, breast cancer consists of two basic types; one that will kill you, and one that will not. In both cases, all the treatment in the world will not affect the outcome. This was highlighted in a post mortem article published by a journalist in the UK and discussed previously in this chapter. The journalist was diagnosed with breast cancer, had it treated (mastectomy, radiation therapy, and chemotherapy) and died of breast cancer 10 years later. While waiting to die, she decided to take on a fantastic challenge. She traveled the world attending as many lectures on breast cancer as possible, and asked the lecturers why she was dying from cancer after she had everything that science had to offer, and after putting her body through serious trauma.

What she found out shocked her and was ignored by most physicians and politicians. The conclusion is what I stated above regarding there being two basic types of breast cancer and their treatability or lack thereof. Sadly, it took an investigative reporter to find a medical truth, not a scientist. She was put through unnecessary treatments which had a huge negative effect on her quality of life.

A more recent article by Peggy Orenstein confirmed the article above.

And so I say, there really is no reason to be examined or treated for breast cancer, as your outcome has nothing to do with treatment. But big government says differently.

The ACA used medical coding in order to win political votes as follows; its authors (democrats) created a coding situation that would win over women. Anything a physician found in a women's breast had to be coded as "breast cancer," including benign tumors and other benign abnormalities. The government did this by forcing physicians to use medical coding defined by the ACA which, of course, the government fabricated.

The tremendous increase in breast cancer diagnosis resulted in two benefits to the ACA. The ACA would get credit for the identification of thousands of cases of breast cancer, and since the majority of whom did not have cancer, the ACA could additionally be touted as having saved countless lives.

This isn't the first time that big government has monkeyed around with healthcare coding. Part of your dental exam includes recording previous dental work, i.e. if you had a filling or crown on tooth #3, we must record it in our computer file. Why? Is it to help you? Is it to better treat you? The correct answer is "none of the above." The real reason for this documentation is for post-mortem identification. IF a body is uncovered that lacks normal ways to identify its owner, such as via facial recognition or fingerprints, as is sometimes that case for someone that has been murdered, and if neither your DNA or fingerprints are on file in any government databases, authorities can often identify you off of your dental records (assuming that enough teeth remain with the corpse). So part of what you are paying for in a dental exam is for the dentist to record something that most likely will never occur and will not benefit you one iota to your dental treatment.

Although this is probably an action that delivers more positive results than negative, the fact that you are not told that you are voluntarily giving big government permission to store information about you is a huge privacy issue. It's only a matter of time before big government will find a similar sneaky way to collect your fingerprints and DNA. (Local police started collecting small children's fingerprints 30 years ago as part of a campaign to help locate your child if they were ever kidnapped or went missing. How much do you want to bet that the FBI has all of this data in their databases?)

And if state or federal money is involved at all in that practice, the dentist has to worry about an inspection of his recordings, so he is forced to comply with this secret collection of personal information.

So what exactly is the Problem?

The problem is YOU!!!!!

Yes, I said YOU. Movie stars become rich by being liked (in some cases, adored) by the public. You like how they act, how they look, how they speak, and the image they create. The fact that they acted according to how they were instructed at Harvard, or that they danced as the masters did had little or nothing to do with what you think of them.

Physicians become rich in the exact same way. Do you like their personality? Do they say what you expect them to say? "We are going to check your blood pressure and cholesterol to be sure your heart is 'healthy' and we will examine you to search for cancer because the earlier you detect it, the easier it is to 'cure' so you can have a long life." Or, "You have to make your husband have regular check-ups also."

As I stated earlier, the object of our book is not to supply the answers to these problems that we have spelled out. Our objective is to make you aware of the many problems that plague our medical and dental systems and to make you aware of why you choose to be part of it. Whether or not you choose to be a customer of the medical industrial complex or to be a free agent is entirely up to you.

We do not KNOW the answer to the many problems we have described here. You must have street smarts in deciding how to live your life. You must learn how to identify correct research and use correct reason. You must learn what is necessary, and what is pop culture. Jerry Lewis raised $2.45 billion through his telethons over 44 years and the Muscular Dystrophy Association is no closer to curing MD. Instead, it has used its power to paint disabled people as "pitiable victims who want and need nothing more than a big charity to take care of or cure them" (as described by disabled rights advocates). These advocates wished that the MDA had spent their time and money on normalizing disabled people through providing accessible transportation and buildings, and by increasing employment opportunities.

We also keep voting our politicians in office and allow them to control us more by convincing us that if you throw enough money at anything, you win the lottery (eternal life). Major illnesses of the world were cured by scientists performing disciplined research, and sometimes having a little luck. Billions of dollars have never cured a major illness, cancer included.

CONCLUSIONS

A BRIEF HISTORY OF MEDICINE
IN THE UNITED STATES

I would like to begin this final section of the book by giving you a brief outline of how I see the history of medicine in the US.

We live in the land of the plenty. Most of the world does not.

Yet....they continue to live.

Our politicians (our government) wants to tell us what to eat in order to live a long (normal) life, as well as what vaccines we must receive, and what medical exams we must have in order to continue to live.

We must keep politicians out of our lives, and out of our bodies.

Let us begin.

The Golden Years

These are years preceding the 1940's. We had greatly advanced our knowledge of what caused most illness and developed most of our surgical procedures which were needed to rehabilitate our injured. Most knowledge was gained from our surgeons treating the victims of our many wars.

We only went to the physician or dentist if our lives depended on it, or were in great pain. The widening use of X-rays meant dentists could attempt to preserve tooth structure before any tooth decay became visually apparent. Or the patient was required to have a badly decayed tooth removed.

The Beginning of Socialized Medicine

World War II brought the awareness of socialism to the US. This belief system was used by politicians to gain power from those who saw themselves as being "left out" of the success others had. As a result, healthcare and dental care were used to bait citizens into voting for socialist minded politicians. The unions were a partner to these extreme left-leaning politicians.

Together, the unions and big government worked to come up with a manipulative system of presenting what those "left out" could have if only they voted to allow government to control a large part of their lives. Medical and Dental Insurance was invented, and misinformation was necessary to "sell" them to the public.

"Look at all these bad things you might have but don't know about because you don't possess medical or dental insurance! Listen to us (the politicians), not the scientists!"

The Current System

Basically what you have read so far in this book.

The Future Medical/Dental System of the US

The Ultra Liberals have been hard at work in the US recently. In 2008, the U.S. voted in a president with obvious socialist views; he was an enemy of the free market and he wanted government to make the most important decisions about the economy. (But Obama is not a true socialist since, outside of nationalizing the healthcare insurance with a single payer solution, he does not want government ownership of the means of production). What Obama wanted most of all was government control of the economy while allowing private ownership of the means of production. His model would allow government to call the shots, but when their policies led to economic failures, they could blame the private sector. Obama was, like most politicians, an excellent salesman who sought power at all costs.

In 2016, 46% of registered Democrats wanted Bernie Sanders, a self-declared Democrat Socialist, to run for president; Hilary Clinton was selected, primarily because the DNC uses super delegates, and the party felt that it was her turn to run.

But the Democratic Party is not alone in its desire for big government, one of the guiding principles of socialism; the Republican Party is also a big fan. Under George W. Bush, federal spending increased 53% (in real terms). And he oversaw No Child Left Behind, Medicare Part D, and bank bailouts. Even Ronald Reagan oversaw an increase in federal spending of 22%. But this was mostly in military spending, which arguably caused the USSR to go bankrupt, putting the final nail in the coffin of Communism.

One of those costs of American politicians spending more of our taxpayer's dollars is your health and wellbeing. There is a big push for politicians (government) to control all of our lives. They campaign for you to give them all your money so that they can decide how to use it on you (or not use it).

Ignorance is the key, and they have a big head start in making us all a lot dumber. Scientists are now hand-picked due to their allegiance to a political party. The internet is their communication instrument, as more and more people worship it rather than the written word. And it is threatening our culture, a culture that was once characterized as one of well carried out research with no agenda other than good science.

It will be "tribal" intellect as scientists will happily make up scientific papers to please the political parties that fund them. We will no longer be treated for ailments. We will receive treatment as cattle do now. They all receive the same immunizations, antibiotics, and food. And you will all receive it, whether you want them or not, whether you benefit or not.

Our great physicians, dentists and other scientists will be lost.

Schools and institutions

Today, medical and dental students got where they were by honing their listening skills, and reading and repeating on multiple choice tests. We did not get into the professional schools by thinking about things, or solving problems. If you put it in terms of evolution, we did not evolve to solve problems and care about patients.

In fact, the education system from high school through dental/medical school is set up to reward those who can come up with the response that their instructors told them to believe, or that their books taught them. It is similar to a dog who begs to get a treat and wags his tail when he does the correct trick. Neither are taught to diagnose and think.

There are a few who do break the mold and turn out to be great physicians and dentists, but they are being squeezed out by these greater forces.

It takes special students to be thinkers and care givers. Why some make this leap, I do not know. I have been treated by very talented professionals who thought outside the box and saw their position as one of increasing their patient's human experience. Unfortunately, I have also been treated or examined by the typical practitioners who only want to spit out what they were taught and to treat patients in order to impress their colleagues with procedures (complicated surgery) or with success (as demonstrated by finances). I have yet to hear a practitioner express their success by how many people's lives they enriched.

As patient/customers, we are just as much to blame because we seem to seek out the "successful" practitioner more defined by how nicely decorated their office is instead of by their abilities to optimize their patient's quality of life. We are influenced by wealth.

And all of this behavior has led to practitioner's closing their minds to alternative principles. I have entered chat rooms concerning medical issues because my physicians were not paying attention to my problems. I learned the most about my conditions from communicating with other patients with similar conditions, not from consultations with physicians.

Interestingly, when I challenged physicians by sharing properly performed research that I discovered about my condition and their cures, I was shunned and banned from the websites. So not only are patients the problem, physicians and dentists are so caught up in proving that they are correct that, when shown truths in research they cannot accept, they close themselves up (nothing to see here).

Cognitive Dissonance Surrounding Healthcare in America

Cognitive dissonance is a state of having inconsistent thoughts, beliefs, or attitudes, especially as relating to behavioral decisions and attitude change. A simple example is when a person that is cheating on their significant other. They rationalize their behavior by saying, "What they don't know won't hurt them." And the majority of Americans believe that government should stay off of our backs, while also believing that government should step in and solve our biggest problems. These are incompatible beliefs; this is another example of cognitive dissonance.

The American practice of Healthcare Gone Wild is based on cognitive dissonance. In FDR's 1944 State of the Union Address, he called for an Economic Bill of Rights, including "the right to adequate medical care and the opportunity to achieve and enjoy good health". This sentiment grew, and by 2016, 60% of Americans believed that government should be responsible for ensuring healthcare coverage for all Americans.

In 2018, Americans spent $2.4 trillion on healthcare, representing 18% of our GDP (Gross Domestic Product). This number should astound you; if the US healthcare industry was its own country, it would be the eighth largest economy in the world! Other developed countries spend between 10 and 12% of GDP. Healthcare spending is higher in the U.S. in the following categories; drug usage rates and prices, medical devices, physician and nurse salaries and, last but not least, administrative costs to process medical claims (source: *Journal of the American Medical Association*).

As stated earlier, the ACA was not designed to reduce healthcare as a percent of GDP, making healthcare more "affordable," it was designed to make health *insurance* more affordable, especially to people not employed, underemployed, or working but without access to employer sponsored health coverage. And despite the ACA being the result of a Democratic controlled Executive and Legislative branches of government working without input from the other party, (but don't forget that Republicans used the same process to stick us with the 2018 tax cut for the rich!), healthcare is slowly becoming an entitlement and a political third rail issue like Social Security, meaning we will never take it away, and that the medical industrial complex will continue to increase profits ad infinitum, and that both parties will continue to accept contributions from the medical industrial complex and their lobbyists, helping them remain in office.

The cognitive dissonance results from this; most of us think that Americans are entitled to healthcare and that the government should do everything to make it happen. But healthcare costs continue to grow as a percent of GDP and are on a trajectory to become unsustainable (33% by 2040, according to a 2015 estimate by the Congressional Budget Office), most likely placing America in a situation where we will require austerity measures. Unless we do something to reduce demand and to control costs, we're on an unstainable path to catastrophe.

GENERAL CONCLUSIONS

What should the role of our healthcare practitioners be?

A short answer to the above is that the role of our medical/dental professionals should be "to better the human experience", or at least that is what most of us think it should be. In reality, very few healthcare practitioners live by that creed.

Most physicians and dentists work on the premise "don't rock the boat," which means they prefer to be "chameleons" and just adapt to do or say what their perceived superiors are doing. They do not search for the "truth" or for better research. Instead, they listen to what others say and repeat what they have heard so that they can fit in and conform.

Preventive medicine does not exist. General practitioners should only act as "emergency room *light*" (aka, walk-in clinics). The only true physicians are emergency room doctors, and the medical and surgical staffs at hospitals that tend to patients admitted after their trip to the ER, or from being diagnosed by their doctor's with a life threatening situation. They practice what medicine was meant to be. Unfortunately, they are subject to the same rules as doctors in private practice, as well as an additional layer of rules that the hospital piles on, so they also have to order unnecessary tests to both avoid malpractice lawsuits and to run up the tab on the customer's visit to their establishment.

And for sure, "preventive" dentistry does not exist. What does exist is "preservation" dentistry. Going to the dentist before something breaks or hurts will preserve tooth structure. The truth is that no matter what a dentist does, they can never return your damaged tooth to its original feel or function.

Government controlled healthcare creates facilities where citizens are treated like animals, like herds of sheep. Citizens are herded into crowded facilities where doctors and dentists are over booked to the point of them wanting to quit. There are so many regulations that

90 percent of the physician's time, energy and thought processes are occupied by a computer program.

You will receive only what the lobbyist groups influencing government officials think is needed based on what they have read on social media, more precisely, what the medical industrial complex wants you to know.

Like sheep which are herded into pastures and lined up for vaccines, you too will be lined up and injected with what the current politician decides is "good" for you. And that will be called "good healthcare for all."

No one wants to be ripped off buying a car with hidden defects, or buying an investment that will surely fail. So why do we want to be ripped off by a doctor or dentist telling us that we need a regular exam or test, or be told that we could get "cancer", or not survive into old age and so we will not see our children grow up. That is exactly what we are being told by pharmaceutical commercials, by our doctors and dentists, and by insurance companies and politicians.

The problem is, those threats of evil things that will happen if we don't adhere to their regimen, are not supported by science. By not performing a medical procedure, a physician or dentist could put their practice into financial ruin. So part of the problem is human nature. Not to get too political, but most of the problem deals with theoretical and practical capitalism and socialism.

Capitalism is a great economic system for allocating resources, especially scarce resources. But, it requires that we all be good consumers, that we act rationally and consume only those goods and services that have value, improving our economic and/or emotional well-being. As consumers, it is up to us to allocate our limited disposable resources (money, time, emotional capital). And guess what; we are *mediocre* consumers, achieving a grade of C or C- at best! We allow marketers to influence our consumption habits versus conducting research and cost justifying our purchases of goods and services, and in the expenditure of our time and emotional capital. Tell me, who really needs a 6,000 pound SUV that is generally only transporting one person 90% of the time and carrying less than a cubic foot of cargo? Does anyone really need a $10,000+ diamond engagement ring that would be only be worth less than $1,000 if DeBeers didn't control the supply of diamonds so tightly? Do any of us receive any long-term benefit from a day of "retail therapy" spent buying stuff to bring us temporary happiness because we don't have the time to spend with friends and family because we're working long hours, or binge watching pointless TV (the average American household watches just under 8 hours per day)? We've turned into W.C. Field and P.T. Barnum's suckers, succumbing to peer pressure and to insane marketing campaigns. And the fact that the unethical capitalists buy off politicians to get away with outright lying to us to trick us into consuming their overpriced and/or over-rated goods and services serves only to fuel the issues between theoretical capitalism and the way capitalism is practiced. But, for all its problems, Capitalism is the best system to enable the best inventors, entrepreneurs and people with talent to be able to rise to the top and create true value to consumers.

Now let's discuss socialism. The downfall of the USSR and Venezuela, the collapse of Cuba's economy, the abject poverty of North Korea, and the governments of China and Vietnam's migration to free market capitalism over state managed economies, are all sufficient evidence of the insufficiencies of socialism as an economic system. And big government just puts one more notch in our county's march to socialism, minimally, along the lines of Western Europe, Canada and Australia. The ACA is not going away anytime soon, and the medical industrial complex will be managed more and more by big government then by free market forces over time, most likely migrating to a single payer system, most likely, universal Medicare. Which is what the Democratic Party envisioned when they created the ACA.

Allow me to provide one example within the medical industrial complex that brilliantly points out the virtues of capitalism over socialism. It involves vision correction with refractive surgery to treat myopia (near-sightedness).

Thirty years ago, if you had to wear corrective lenses, you could fork over $15,000 and undergo the radial keratotomy process, where the corneas were reshaped using scalpel incisions. The process had a high success rate at improving the patient's vision and not making them blind, but, it could only be performed once, and it didn't always allow the patient to rid themselves of corrective lenses.

A decade or so later, along comes LASIK surgery, an exponentially safer and superior technology, allowing most of its patients to eliminate corrective lenses, and not because it made them blind! In 2016, the cost of LASIK was down to around $5,000 for both eyes. So in less than two decades, the demand for refractive surgical correction of myopia led to a significant improvement in results (minimally, twice as good of an output result), and at least a 60% reduction in cost.

And this was all done via the free market; almost all of the procedures were paid for by the patient, since almost no insurers covered the procedure!

So now we suffer from a hybridization of capitalism and socialism. We suffer because we generally get the worst of both systems. TV, radio and internet commercials constantly tell us to "ask your physician" about product X. Or find out if you can control your symptoms better with product Y. The medical industrial complex has just benefited from big government by providing them with another 30 million customers, making their marketing campaigns even that much more effective; their message was already going out to the 30 million, but they didn't care when they weren't a customer!

Our symptoms are now abbreviated as the medical and pharmaceutical companies think that you can only be convinced to go to your doctor if you are not embarrassed by saying what ails you.

All of this is geared up to convince the public that they NEED things. We no longer go to the dentist or doctor to repair us. We now go because we think we are supposed to search for these symptoms we see in the media and that we must have them corrected, especially if our insurance pays for it!

Most of us think that since we are paying for insurance, we must get whatever we can out of it, whether we need it or not. And our physicians and dentists are happy to oblige.

Just try to get a doctor or dental appointment in December to be able to take advantage of the fact that your insurance co-pay has been met!

One last thought on the need to not allow the US to adopt a state run healthcare system like the rest of the industrial world. The US accounts for 57% of all new chemical entities (pharmaceuticals) in the 2000's, up from 31% in the 1970's. The US has 93 Nobel Prizes in

Physiology and Medicine, nearly half. And in terms of publications in biology and medicine, 40% come from the US.

Socialized medicine is bound to reduce the output from US innovators, as it has done in the industrialized nations currently practicing it.

Just because it can be done doesn't mean it should be done

Dr. Norman Hadler said it best; "Our institutions are training our physicians to perform many great surgical procedures. Problem is, they are performing these procedures when they should not."

Kidneys stones. Over ten percent of Americans have experienced at least one. Painful. But what do ALL urologists tell us? "Be sure to use this sieve and collect the stone so we can analyze it and tell you what not to eat." The idea is that you only get kidney stones if you are eating or drinking substances that causes them. I have yet to read one single report or research paper demonstrating that the knowledge of what makes the stone up has prevented one kidney stone.

Removing body parts of cancer patients (breasts, prostates, faces) when the patient winds up with a worse quality of life is not a success. To a physician, it is. They can hold their chest out, thinking they saved a life. They can impress their friends and neighbors with a new car in the driveway.

What does the poor patient have to show?

Perhaps a patient will feel vindicated in using up their time with their family by going to the physicians over the years in a search for cancer. They feel justified. They feel they were right. They knew they had cancer and they just had to search long enough to find it. Now they have no retirement savings, they've lost precious time they could have devoted to raising their children, and they can't enjoy retirement anyway, now lacking bowel control, or some other missing body part. But they were "right." They might ridicule their friends for not going to regular medical exams and not having every test that exists done to them.

After age 75, even if your doctor finds something at your 6 month check-ups, or you simply find something that society wants you to correct, think twice before you correct it! Especially if it is cancer. Physicians incorrectly behave as if they have failed if a patient dies. ALL of us will die. If you give this predicament some serious thought, you will most likely conclude that It is better for your quality of life if you and your physician accept this and do not continue to be treated for every illness or body change that occurs as a result of being alive "just because" you can.

Physicians want you to think your life is a "whack a mole" game

Whack a mole, my favorite childhood arcade game. A problem (the mole) pops up and you hit it. It goes away, but another problem (another mole) pops up and, you attempt to hit it. If you manage to hit enough moles fast enough, you win.

What if the moles represented illness? One is cancer, one is high blood pressure, and one is diabetes?

Physicians promote their trade as helping you win at whack a mole.

Physicians must stop supporting their juvenile beliefs over real science. They must go back to being scientists that practice the science of medicine.

Politicians must cease their unbridled seeking of power at the cost of their constituent's diminished human experience.

Physicians must stop hiding costs. Hospitals and physicians both exist in a "universe" of being above everyone else, and believe that all of us "mere" patients must accept whatever they say, and to pay whatever they state, never knowing the total cost until after you are treated.

I can remember trips to the doctor's office as a child. When you arrived, there were one or two other patients in the waiting room. The doctor's office had one additional person working with them, and that person was usually a nurse who also greeted patients, made appointments, and handled the minimal amount of paperwork required at that time. You went straight to see the doctor, not to another waiting room. And best of all, the doctor knew your name without looking at your chart! The doctor listened to you, spent time not only learning what ailed you, but got to know you as a person.

Today, you are a customer and the doctor's office is a place of business, with a dozen people assembled in the reception area, and another three or four in smaller waiting rooms. The practice has two employees in the reception area, making appointments, processing paperwork, and running the office on a day to day basis, and an office manager comes and goes, overseeing this operation. There are probably a pair of nurses taking your vital signs and getting a perfunctory explanation of what is ailing you, then pulling your chart so they can let the doctor know your name, because they have five to ten times more patients and can't possibly take the time to know your name unassisted.

In 2014, a general practitioner made an average of $220,000 per year in the U.S. In 1982, they made $80,000, which is worth $215,000 in 2014 dollars.

And they call this progress.

Dentists

Those 4 out of 5 dentists were paid to attend a seminar on a product, then asked if they recommend it to their patients. Of course they will say "yes" since they just received a free paid vacation by the company.

This is a big problem. I have been closed out of three forums on social media, all dealing with physicians or dentists. When I challenged them with questions such as, "Is there any research that demonstrates the value of lowering a patient's blood pressure?", or if I stated that there was no evidence that anything can prevent colitis, and while attempting to present the research to the audience, I was "banned" from the forums for violating their policy of "politeness." Is that what we are all doing now? Are we not supposed to speak if it hurts someone's feelings?

The problem is that dentists and physicians have fallen into the trap of doing what others do, rather than doing what the science proves. Their social presence trumps correctness. They surely will not be criticized if they kill a patient as long as they did what their colleagues said to do.

A dentist's desire to treat patients in a true and caring way has been hijacked by the dental supply companies, who have ingeniously convinced them that all that ails a patient can be cured by constant gum treatments and an electric tooth brush.

The dental supply companies named this the "soft tissue program" and encouraged the dentists to communicate this to their patients. They are told if you do not offer this treatment to patients, you are not offering the best that dentistry can supply and therefore you are committing malpractice.

The same occurs with bone grafts for simple tooth extractions and intraoral cancer exams, both of which have been proven to not be necessary: the cancer exams have proven to not prevent cancer at all, nor to provide better outcomes from cancer treatment.

A military pilot does not ask a friend what to do in a situation. He asks the instructors who have access to the test pilot results.

In dental schools, I have observed a disturbing pattern of the schools using monetary successful instructors rather than research or practice successful instructors. So instructors treat the students as a colleague and say what they think the student wants to hear.

Mental Health Practitioners

Mental health practitioners have failed us. Their first misstep happened in the 1960's, when psychiatric drugs became available to treat schizophrenia and depression. While this was a much better way to treat patients with major mental illnesses (especially over being confined to mental institutes and being jolted with electroconvulsive therapy), the market soon flooded with meds to be used to treat the general population, leading to a situation where, by 2004, over 50% of households had someone seek mental health treatment, with one in six Americans taking some form of psychiatric drug by 2016 (antidepressants were most common, followed by anxiety relievers and antipsychotics). These practitioners have become pill pushers, medicating us, sometimes getting us addicted, instead of forcing us to deal with our issues. And why? As we've already determined, they have gone from primarily using clinical data covering thousands of patients to using personal and peer experience covering a limited sample size.

The Medical Industrial Complex

But the real culprit is our healthcare infrastructure, that part of the medical industrial complex that is driving these failed practices, namely, big pharma, medical and dental schools, medical and dental suppliers, insurance companies, and the most offensive, their partner in crime, big government.

Big pharma manipulates drug pricing and influences both medical professionals and their customers (us!) with their slick marketing tricks.

Medical and dental schools both limit the number of practitioners to keep supply down, while their graduates drive up demand via the learnings they are imparted with from these institutions (not to mention the influence of medical and dental suppliers, insurance companies and government on driving up demand), all of which are guaranteed to drive up prices. It's Economics 101!

Medical and Dental suppliers push products that maximize their profits, supported by invalid research.

Insurance companies encourage poor practices, forcing healthcare practitioners to do unnecessary or impractical procedures, as well as deny treatment in order to reduce costs if they believe they have a good chance of getting away with it, even if it kills the patient/customer!

And what more can be said about big government and the role that they have played in the metamorphosis to the wildness that healthcare demonstrates today? Sure, some of their policies might have been actually designed to help *we the people* that put them in power. But now it's all just a power grab to keep them getting re-elected and to continue the drive to universal healthcare and the potential bankrupting of America. Or worse, once we adapt universal healthcare forces, we will have to ration healthcare. England's National Health Service has been rationing for decades, whether it's denying treatments costing over £30,000 (about $38,000) per QALY (Quality Adjusted Life Years), a measurement of how a treatment extends both the patient's life and improves the quality of their life; aka, death panels, to reducing IVF treatments from 3 to 1 and only then for females meeting their extremely strict eligibility requirement, to limiting non urgent surgery for obese patients and smokers. And all of a sudden you've given big government the ultimate control; they're deciding who gets to live, and for how long.

The Physician's Role in Our Lives

Hundreds of years ago, a physician was primarily handling broke-fix it situations and was the last resort to save an ill or injured person's life. They were not trained as there was no references, no information, on what to do or how to heal a person.

As late as the 1920's, our government put out publications on health. They dealt with how to remedy a condition; how to stop pain, like *Health Through Natural Methods by* Edwin J. Ross. Medicine had nothing to do with prevention.

Not until the 1940's did our society attach the word "preventative" to the term medicine. And this was introduced via corporations reacting to big government wage freezes, followed by unions with political agendas, in the form of health insurance.

Health insurance initially had an adverse impact on physicians in two ways, both involving an increase in paperwork. The first was a change in their cash flow, from receiving cash payment to billing patients and/or their insurance, the second, paperwork documentation accompanying a patient visit. In order to make this a win-win situation for big government, unions and physicians, preventative medical exams occurring annually or twice per year were invented. This was enacted for dentists not long afterwards. Suddenly, everybody's happy. And everybody's getting wealthier. Placating to someone's greed goes a long way to appease a lot of problems!

So, you see, the need for annual or semi-annual check-up was never based on medical information or studies. They were simply based on politics and greed.

Dr. Norman Halder stated that the physician's only role should be emergency care, such as stopping bleeding, or setting a broken leg. There is no such thing as preventive medicine.

The role of medicine is to train skilled physicians who can repair us in times of emergency. Their role is not to attempt to be god and predict what will kill you and to try and stop it from occurring. We all will die. Some will die of cancer, others of cardiovascular disease, and others yet from brain disease. Some will die of time. But we will all die.

There is a limit to a human life span. Human longevity has not been lengthened at all for as long as scientists can determine. We have identified through examinations of prehistoric skeletons and early European records, that ancient humans lived to be over 100 years old. All that modern science has done for humans has allowed more of us to live longer than 30 years, mostly with the use of vaccines and extreme surgeries, and treatments that perhaps should not have been done.

So now our physicians give in to political correctness, mass media and the medical industrial complex, treating society's fears, not the patient's physical injuries. They treat emotions, and apparently that is what our misinformed and/or uneducated population wants, because they demand it, and someone else pays for it, indirectly, through insurance.

If indeed the physicians are correct in telling us we must be tested regularly in order to lengthen our lives, why don't they simply perform every test known to us immediately after we are born, and then every month afterwards for our entire life?

Does the above just seem too insane? Or is it already in the works? Perhaps this is what big government is aiming at. No one could possibly afford to have all these tests run every month. Big government will eventually use this to gain your support in funding all-inclusive insurance. They will create the problem that only they can solve.

Just because it can be done doesn't mean it should be done

You are 85 years old. You are in a hospital bed with congestive heart failure and pneumonia.

You have Medicare, a government run health insurance plan. Your physician is thorough and orders a full dental and cancer screening. The results of the exams uncover skin cancer on your arm, and an abscessed tooth, neither of which bothers you.

What will your physician tell you? What should he tell you? What will he do as a result of you having a government insurance policy versus paying cash?

Other physicians have addressed this conundrum in published works. Their protocol would determine the nature of the life threatening situation, the congestive heart failure and pneumonia. It would determine if the patient was strong enough for each form of treatment, given their advanced age and poor state of well-being. Most likely, the patient would die from any type of surgery, so it would be avoided. The patient could be treated primarily for pneumonia, and be discharged with a treatment plan focusing on making them comfortable, primarily through breathing treatment and pain medication. The patient's relatives could also opt to have nothing done to the patient.

The skin cancer and abscessed tooth would probably be ignored, given the low probability that either condition would advance to a point to require treatment before the patient died from old age. Sadly, this protocol is not in agreement with what our current healthcare system prescribes. I and others agree that our medical organizations should be focused on "quality of life", and not on "do whatever is possible to remove any diseased condition no matter what the outcome, in order to protect yourself against being sued."

Continuing with the above situation, the medical industrial complex would look at you as a customer. A great customer. They would order countless tests to update the status of your heart. They would pump you full of antibiotics and hook you up to an IV drip. Hopefully, they could get you into their Intensive Care Unit, converting you from a Silver to Gold status customer. Once your lungs are healthy enough for surgery, they'll talk you into angioplasty to open up your arteries, or heart valve repair, or the granddaddy of all surgeries, a heart-lung transplant! But given your advanced age and poor state of well-being, even the most unethical physicians wouldn't dare recommend it. However, you can still achieve Platinum customer status; you have cancer! While they are treating your pneumonia, they'll deal with the abscessed tooth and start staging your cancer, working up treatment options, which may include surgery, radiation therapy and/or chemotherapy, or maybe (if they're lucky and you're not) all three! Minimally, they'll get you on more ACE Inhibitors, beta-blockers and diuretics for the bad ticker, and immunotherapy drugs to fight the cancer.

An 85 year old person is at their end of their life, or close to it. If you will not be leaving the hospital alive, why treat you for something that won't kill you for another 20 years? Or remove a tooth that is not causing a problem but the actions of removing it can cause psychological and physical stress?

I would consider a physician/dentist who wanted to perform the above procedures on a patient in the above circumstance to be committing malpractice and undue harm and suffering to a patient who would not benefit from these procedures.

Unfortunately, our legal system does not feel this way.

Hope?

This book does not offer solutions to the problems discussed herein, however, we have found hope in one new and exciting approach to practicing medicine area.

Online physicians groups have started up. I have used them. My group focused on actually helping me, the PATIENT (not their customer), instead of pushing unnecessary tests. A follow-up appointment three months after initial treatment is not needed. You do not have to take time off from work to attend face to face appointments with a physician.

You simply text the group, pay a very small fee, and they text you back with questions, speak with you over the phone if needed, and offer solutions within minutes. I received a prescription I needed for my ulcerative colitis in one hour; other physicians would not write the prescription unless I visited their office, then subjected myself to repeated colonoscopies, all of which are unnecessary.

Why must a patient sit face to face with a physician in order to renew a prescription? Why can't this be done by text? Or Skype?

Why must a patient take a day off from work after waiting three months for an appointment in order to have their problem addressed?

We have accepted that our lives will be disrupted by doctor appointments, that we must miss work, travel great distances, and subject ourselves to referrals to specialists for expensive and unnecessary tests in order for the doctor to save face.

Finally, there is a vehicle that works for the patients. I hope I am correct and this is the answer to our many problems in the near future.

WARNINGS

Beware....

...of Dr. "Scope", the physician who wants to perform endoscopies or colonoscopies on you for a simple consultation. These procedures bring in big money for the medical office and the physicians think that it is good info for them to record in your chart in case you ever sue them, but provides little information which will allow them to treat your symptoms. They are invasive and potentially dangerous procedures; patients have died from having the procedure performed on them.

These physicians justify performing these procedures on you by saying, "What if you have cancer?"

Beware...

...of Dr. "Moonbeam". These doctors think all can be cured "naturally" by diet or exercise. On one hand, I agree with non-intrusive treatments, but they seem to overdo it and ignore medicines or treatments which might increase your quality of life.

Beware...

...of the follower of fads syndrome. These doctors and dentists think they win accolades and respect among their colleagues if they are offering the latest thing (fad, internet promoted treatment, vitamin, diet). They think they saved your life and that they now will not be sued by the patient due to their being "socially and politically correct".

They justify the expense, both financial and emotional, of the patient by using the above rationale.

There is in fact no data showing that searching for something such as a cancer will prolong your life more than the patient noticing something is wrong with them and then seeking help. It is simply bio plausible and politically correct.

Beware...

...of supporters of old beliefs. These physicians would rather support their old beliefs they learned when they were young than override them and treat you with something that might benefit you. Or worse, they treat you as they were treated when young and deny you correct and tested newer treatments.

Beware...

...of consensus seekers. These dentists, physicians and mental healthcare practitioners decide on what diagnosis to give you, or on what treatment to give you, based on what they think their colleagues would do. It is a social thing. They do not know how to judge research, so they "ask" their drinking buddy and treat you based on what their buddy says.

Fear Mongering

PRE-diabetes.

PRE high blood pressure.

Do you have the urge to urinate?

Our physicians and the medical institutions have been turned into sales persons.

Do any of the fear statements above ring a bell? I am sure they do. And they all have nothing to do with health. They are simply phrases the institutions have placed into the public eye in hopes of shackling you and forcing you to spend more of your emotional capitol on the medical professions.

Being alive is a cause of any condition that can be named. And more of these conditions do not take anything away from your quality of life.

We all experience a juvenile, teenage, adult and senile life stages. Your body will act and feel differently during all these stages. That is nature, and that is the human experience. You can greet all the stages with open arms and enjoy them, or you can succumb to the politicians and institutions and use your emotional and financial capitol on them.

You have the freedom to decide even if social media says you do not.

The Internet and Electronic Records are Making us all Dumber

Electronic files. I have not come across any physician or dentist who thinks electronic or computer patient records are a good thing. And it's even worse if a physician works for a government agency.

Humans work best when they have a tactile connection to their work and ideas (paper). Electronic files have separated the clinicians from this.

I would like to attempt to give you an analogy of the problem using American football as an example:

Your favorite team is on the field. Your team has the ball. You don't have the best players but you do have the most inclusive team judged by the media, you have all nationalities, religions, sexes and sizes of people on your team. Not the best as that would be politically incorrect, and the word "best" might offend some.

A group of government employees designed your play calling computer program. Before the game, the quarterback, followed by the rest of the team, must check in with the computer.

The ball is hiked to the quarterback. He can only throw the ball to his right side wide receiver because the computer program told him to, even though he would be better off by looking over the entire field and finding another receiver, or handing the ball off to a halfback.

Your team loses the game. The players complain that they could play better if they did not have to follow the computer program, but all teams are told they must use this program. They are not allowed to draw plays on paper as it cannot be recorded for government inspectors to see what plays they choose during the game.

Instead of winding down and reviewing what went wrong and relaxing, each member of the team must sign into the computer again and go thru 20 pages of questions, such as, "Did you warm up before the game, yes/no?"

"Did you use the proper shoes and clothes for the game, yes/no?"

Etc.

The players could have learned from their experience of what they were allowed to do and still follow the computer program. They complain to the administrator who runs the computer program that it takes up their valuable time, and that the questions are not pertinent to what they are doing on the field.

The administrator is not an athlete and therefore does not understand why you are complaining. He only responds by stating that the questions are there and you must complete all of them each game in case an attorney tries to sue the team for not preparing correctly, or in case of injury, or a complaint from a fan concerning proper attire.

I hope you can now see what the medical and dental professions go through due to government interference.

Government agencies are run by politicians, or civil servants that ultimately report to politicians, not to business professionals. Most of these agencies are strapped with inefficient bureaucratic policies and practices that have to be overly politically correct; they have a tendency to be highly inefficient and to attract employees that are not risk takers, and that like routine. And these are the people who implement policies developed by politicians, without the benefit of expert testimony in a thorough committee process. No wonder the results are such a bad product.

No wonder we are getting Healthcare Gone Wild!

For example: Unambitious, conceptually minded, politically correct government employees decide what will be in the program. They decide what the physician must answer. All of the boxes must be checked.

At least there is some good news coming from our stupefying internet. It provides a tool for patients to share their experiences on treatments on various medical conditions. They can describe what physicians told them and the treatments they received and what worked for them. I have used it to a great extent and in more than one situation, I gained valuable information while participating in forums on my condition that many physicians did not share with me.

The only problem, I was banned from three forums, from physicians and dentists as they cannot tolerate anyone who presents differing data than what they want to hear. Rather than challenging me to explain myself, or themselves presenting data to show why they had their views, they simply turned me off. This practice is common with politicians blinded by their party's ideology, and unfortunately, this practice is considered to be acceptable by physicians and dentists

I found helpful ways to better my symptoms on other sites.

I think it would be a good idea for physicians to read consumer reviews on treatments they prescribe to their patients.

WHAT DEFINITELY DOES NOT WORK

1. **Routine exams** Study after study has shown that routine exams rarely prevent anything. They might find something that will adversely affect your life, but finding it before you notice symptoms does not make for a better outcome. Additionally, they will find things that will not adversely affect your life (false positives), and that will increase your anxiety and prevent you from enjoying a full life.

   Studies of long-lived humans showed that access to medical care was not a determinant of their longer life.

2. **Vitamins** Studies have shown that patients who take daily vitamins and do not have a deficiency due to a medical problem (such as an absorption deficiency) will die sooner than if they had not taken vitamins routinely.

3. **Blood pressure and cholesterol adjustments** Manipulating these does not affect how long you will live nor will they decrease your chances of heart attack or stroke.

4. **Physical activity** Long term studies and observations demonstrate that people engaged in physically demanding jobs have an 18% greater risk of dying early. There is no optimal amount of exercise for mental and cardiovascular well-being. Our cells can only perform a certain amount of biochemical processes. The more we eat and exert, the faster we use up these finite amounts of processes that our cells are capable of.

5. **Dental cancer screenings** Same as routine medical exams. Studies show that a dentist will not find a cancer before you notice a change in your mouth or throat.

6. **Designing diets to live longer** No combination of foods has been known to increase longevity. All talk of this is based on fads and politics. Milk is not bad for you. Vegetable fat is not better than animal fat in your diet.

7. **Cholesterol** There is no need to check your cholesterol level. Altering this does not benefit anyone.
8. **Alcohol and tobacco** Their use does not guarantee an early death.
9. **Radiation** Radiation does not and never has caused cancer in any animal, including humans.

WHAT DOES WORK

1. **Dental restorations** Removing dental decay early preserves tooth structure and increases tooth longevity.
2. **Periods of starvation** This has been observed to prolong life in non-human studies and suggested in the life histories of long-lived humans. Additionally, this has been proven to reverse type I and type II diabetes in humans.
3. **Lack of concern for things that can kill you** Many centenarians included in their daily routine the use of coffee and tobacco and a lack of modern sanitary conditions. A recent look at the Japanese found that the survivors of the Hiroshima and Nagasaki nuclear bomb explosions have an average life span of over 82 years. Politicians with an agenda would try to convince us this is due to their diet, but science and data shows this is due to exposure to radiation. Radiation kills cancer as proven by decades of radiation therapy. They turned out to have fewer cases of breast cancer than those who did not receive radiation exposure to the breasts.
4. **Emergency care** After all, this is what modern medicine was until big government and unions started exploiting medical insurances. If you break a bone, if you can't stop bleeding, if you have severe pain, go to the hospital or walk-in clinic. You want to be able to have a good quality of life. Scheduled exams do not reduce your chances of having an emergency.
5. **Catastrophic health insurance** High deductible policies are relatively inexpensive and would allow life-saving procedures without bankrupting an individual, and without bankrupting the US economy (as will be the case with Universal Medicare).

CAUSES OF CONFUSION

1. **Loss of peer review of research papers** Medical schools have been studying the amount of research papers that are actually *real* research papers and were alarmed both in the US and Europe at the amount of research published in which the research could not be duplicated, which is the most important aspect of a research project! To have your colleagues read your paper and, from your description of what you did, reproduce the experiment and come up with the same results as the original researcher is the best way to validate research.

    Additionally, these papers were now being published in sleazy journals that identified themselves as medical journals but are merely vehicles for the medical industrial complex to advertise to existing and new customers, both we "patients" and to other members of the complex. The publishers were not performing peer reviews of the papers to determine that the authors followed sound scientific methods in conducting and communicating their research.

2. **Money and politics** Capitalism is the best system the world has known, but recently the medical field has been sacrificing patient care in the name of profit. Socialism is the most damaging political system known, and it sacrifices medical care in order to get votes and to control citizens.

3. **Social media (including television)** Most of us have become accustomed to hearing soundbites and reading one-liners about everything and everyone. We believe what we hear and see and we want it now. If a friend repeats something you saw, you take it as fact. Physicians and dentists are no different. They will practice what they see and believe it to be true without questioning its validity based on science, and they will deliver what their audience (their patients) want. It is a cycle of the ignorant giving in to the ignorant.

EVERYTHING HAS A
BEGINNING AND AN END

Including us.

Including this book.

All humans, in fact, ALL animals and plants that we know of, have a beginning, a longer middle age time, and a dying act.

John Gribbin (*In The Beginning*) very clearly and convincingly describes the multiverse (all that exists, even if we can't detect it). The universe came from nothing and expansion has allowed for many things to form (the entire universe, including galaxies, stars, planets, life forms, including us).

They ALL have a beginning and an end, including us. We cannot prevent this "end" from occurring no matter how much searching we perform for "cancer."

As stated earlier, physicians should be aiding us in dealing with this inevitable end, and must not see it as a failure on their part. This would prevent them from suggesting unnecessary procedures, exams and drugs to us simply because we are experiencing normal life.

OUR ADVICE

Consider your physician to be only a choice of last resort. You broke your leg, you feel sick and want it to stop, you are bleeding and it won't stop.

Physicians should keep you alive in an emergency, or correct a major abnormality. There is no reason to go to a doctor's office in the misbelief that this practice will allow you will to live longer or to prevent pain.

Consume food and drinks that you like. Participate in activities that you like. Experiment with new things.

Live your life, consuming experiences with your friends and family, not being brainwashed into leading a life thinking you can sacrifice your emotional, monetary or time capitol in order to gain immortality.

Time to say good bye. We hope you have enjoyed our show.

RX: One cigar a week, one drink a day

Have a happy life.

REFERENCES

High Blood Pressure Myths and Lies-published on Primal Diet, Modern Health, May 9, 2018

Your Annual Physical Wastes Time, Money, Some Doctors Say, Kim Pastor, *USA Today*, Jan 31, 2016

The Vitamin Myth: Why We Think We Need Supplements, Paul Offit, *The Atlantic*, July 19, 2013

Does Treating High Blood Pressure Do Any Good?, Dr. Malcolm Kendrick, *drmalcolmkendrick.org*, April, 2, 2012.

Understanding Why, Evolution, Beliefs, and Your Reality, George F. Naryshkin August, 2004

god is not Great, Christopher Hitchens, May 2007

Malay Archipelago, Volumes 1 and 2, Alfred Russel Wallace, 1869

Beta Blockers are Busted-What Happens Next?, Josh Bloom, *New Scientist*, November 7, 2012

HEALTH Through Natural Methods, Edwin J. Ross, *he American Health Association*, 1924

Healthy? Says Who?, Dr. George F. Naryshkin February, 2014

The Last Well Person, Nortin M. Hadler M.D., 2004

When Evidence Says No, but Doctors Say Yes, David Epstein and Propublica, The *Atlantic*, February 22, 2017

Is Lead Shielding Needed to Protect Pregnant Patients?, Tony Edwards, Ed in Chief, *Dental News*, September 22, 2015

Do we really live longer than our ancestors?, Amanda Ruggeri, *BBC.com*, October 3, 2018

Does Radiation Really Cause Cancer? Conversation among Professionals, John Adams, *Atomic Insights*, January 18, 2012

Antimicrobial Resistance of Staph Aureus and oral streptococci strains from high -risk endocarditis patients, Grupo, et al, *General Dentistry*, June 3, 2005.

Leukemia incidence of 96,000 atomic bomb survivors is compelling evidence that the LNT model is wrong, Jerry M. Cutler, *Arch Toxic*, January 24, 2014

Radiation Unlikely to be responsible for the high cancer rates among distal Hiroshima A-bomb Survivors- Grant, et al, *Environmental Health Prev Med*, April 8, 2009,

Does Periodontitis cause heart disease?, Mattila, *European Heart Journal*, December 1, 2003

A survey of pain, pressure, and discomfort by Commonly Used Oral Local Anesthesia Injections, Kaufman, et al, *Anesthesia Progress*, January 30, 2004

What Causes Heart Disease part forty-eight, Dr. Malcolm Kendrick, *drmalcolmkendrick.org*, March 22, 2018

Conversation by phone with the Florida Dept of Radiation, Oct 2014.

Radiation Protection and Lead Aprons, Norman Medins DDS, *Art of Dentistry*, February 21, 2014

Clinical Psychology Review 33 (2013) p. 885, Scott Liliesfeld, Lorie Ritschel, Stephen Jay, Lynn Robin Cautin, Robert Latzman

Comparison of Mortality and Comorbidity Rates Between Holocaust Survivors and Individuals in the General Population in Israel, Naama Fund, MSc1 (Nachman Ash, MD; Avi Porath, MD; Varda Shalev, MD; Gideon Koren, MD), *JAMA,* January 5, 2019

The US has a lot of money, but it does not look like a developed country, Annalisa Merelli, *Quartz,* March 10, 2017

Stem cell divisions, somatic mutations, cancer etiology, and cancer prevention, Cristian Tomasetti, Lu Li, Bert Vogelstein, *Science,* March 24, 2017

The contribution of cytotoxic chemotherapy to 5-year survival in adult malignancies, G. Morgan, R. Ward, M. Barton, *Clinical Oncology,* December 16, 2004

Neoadjuvant chemotherapy induces breast cancer metastasis through a TMEM-mediated mechanism, George S. Karagiannis, Jessica M. Pastoriza, Yarong Wang, Allison S. Harney, *Science Translation Medicine,* July 5, 2017

Does 'bad' cholesterol deserve its bad name?, Ana Sandoiu, *Medical News Today,* October 2, 2018

Misclassification of cardiometabolic health when using body mass index categories in NHANES 2005–2012, A J Tomiyama, J M Hunger, J Nguyen-Cuu & C Wells, *International Journal of Obesity,* February 4, 2016

Can You Be Overweight and Still Be Healthy?, Monica Reinagel, *Scientific America,* July 31, 2013

Human helminth therapy to treat inflammatory disorders- where do we stand?, Helena Helmby, *US National Library of Medicine* (National Institute of Heath), 2015 Mar 26.

Extreme high high-density lipoprotein cholesterol is paradoxically associated with high mortality in men and women: two prospective cohort studies, Christian M. Madsen, Anette Varbo, Børge G. Nordestgaard, *European Heart Journal*, Volume 38, Issue 32, August 21, 2017.

Physically demanding jobs may raise risk of early death, study finds, Steven Reinberg, *HealthDay*, May 15, 2018

25-Year Physical Activity Trajectories and Development of Subclinical Coronary Artery Disease as Measured by Coronary Artery Calcium: The Coronary Artery Risk Development in Young Adults (CARDIA) Study, Deepika R. Laddu, Jamal S. Rana, Rosenda Murillo, Michael E. Sorel, Charles P. Quesenberry Jr., Norrina B. Allen, Kelley P. Gabriel, Mercedes R. Carnethon, Kiang Liu, Jared P. Reis, Donald Lloyd-Jones, J. Jeffrey Carr, Stephen Sidney, *Mayo Clinic Proceedings*, November 2017.

Antimicrobial Resistance: Tackling a crisis for the health and wealth of nations, Jim O'Neil, *The Review on Antimicrobial Resistance*, December 2014

Are antibiotics turning livestock into superbug factories?, Giorgia Guglielmi, *Science*, September 28, 2017

Big Pharma games the System to make generic drugs more expensive, Emma Court, *Market Watch*, August 3, 2018

How the U.S. Pays 3 Times More for Drugs, Ben Hirschler, *Scientific America*, 2019

Cervical artery dissection related to chiropractic manipulation: One institution's experience, Kennell, Daghfal, Patel, DeSanto, Waterman, Bertino, *University of Illinois College of Medicine, Journal of Family Practice*, September 2017

Psychiatric Axis I Comorbidities among Patients with Gender Dysphoria, Mazaheri Meybodi, Hajebi, Ghanbari Jolfaei, *US National Library of Medicine National Institutes of Health*, August 11, 2014

A Review of the Opioid Epidemic: What Do We Do About It? Shipton EA, Shipton EE, Shipton AJ, *Pain and Therapy*, June 2018.

Looking for Evidence That Therapy Works, Harriet Brown, *Well Magazine*, March 25, 2013

Bad Medicine: How the AMA Undermined Primary Care in America, Brian Klepper, *Wall Street Journal*, December 13, 2007

Aging Is Reversible—at Least in Human Cells and Live Mice, Karen Weintraub, *Scientific America*, December 15, 2016

Obama is Not a Socialist, Thomas Sowell, *Capital Magazine*, May 31, 2014

Our Feel-Good War on Breast Cancer, Peggy Orenstein, *The New York Times Magazine*, April 25, 2013

Prostate Cancer MRI scans to be introduced after pilot, Owain Clarke, *BBC News*, December 12, 2018

Very Large Amounts of Radiation are Required to Produce Cancer, Antone L Brooks, et al, *Dose-Response* September 30, 2007

The 50 Most Important Life-Saving Breakthroughs in History, Jeff Desjardins, *AperionCare*, March 26, 2018

The Food Guide Pyramid: Will the Defects Be Corrected?, A. Ottoboni, *Journal of the American Physicians and Surgeons*, November, 2004

Which Countries Excel in Creating New Drugs? It's Complicated, Stewart Lyman, *Xconomy*, 2 November 2014

Centers for Medicare &Medicaide Services, The Centrer for Information and Insurance Oversight, pub on CMS.gov, not dated

We are being screwed over by our health-care system, and it's all our fault!

Did you know?

- High blood pressure did not exist as a medical diagnosis until pharmaceutical companies invented medicines that can lower it and convinced physicians to sell it to their patients.
- There are two kinds of breast cancer: one that will kill you no matter what you do and one that won't. Yet a breast cancer diagnosis will have your physicians ready to cut you open, radiate you, and pump chemicals into your body—all so they can "save" you.
- The health-care industry, aka the medical industrial complex, is the largest industry in the US and is doing everything they can to make you a lifelong customer. And they are in bed with big government to stay no. 1.

How did America get itself into this mess? Well, we, the people, are partly to blame!

- We don't question our physicians, consuming their "cures" to make us live longer and fix all our problems with a simple pill or procedure.
- We buy into the media's reinforcement of the above solutions.
- And we allow our politicians to take money from the medical industrial complex to get reelected while making the health-care industry the fourth largest economy on earth!

Do you want to live the life you deserve—enjoying your friends, family, and hobbies? Or do you want to deplete your emotional and financial capital and your time bank worrying about every little thing that the media, the government, and your physicians say can kill you? If you answered yes to the former question, read *Healthcare Gone Wild*. (If you answered yes to the latter, you should read *Healthcare Gone Wild* immediately; stop living in fear and depriving yourself of happiness now!)

CPSIA information can be obtained
at www.ICGtesting.com
Printed in the USA
BVHW030026140819
555828BV00001B/11/P

9 781728 319049